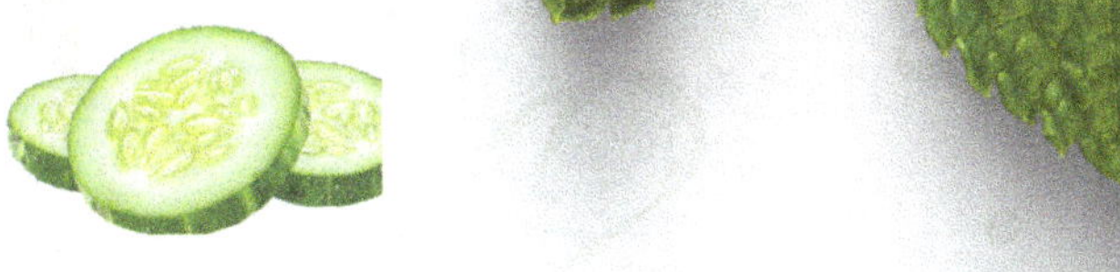

THE COMPLETE

GERD

2024 EDITION

Delicious Recipes with Full-Color Pictures, Dietary Info for Managing Acid Reflux

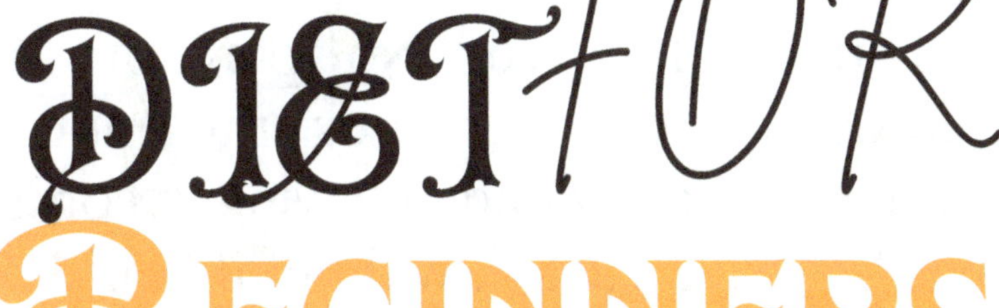

DIET FOR BEGINNERS

VAKARE RIMKUTE

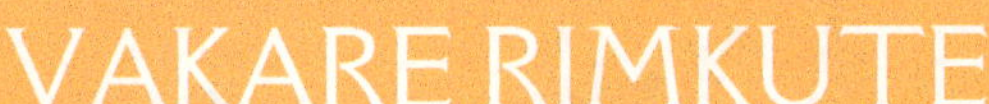

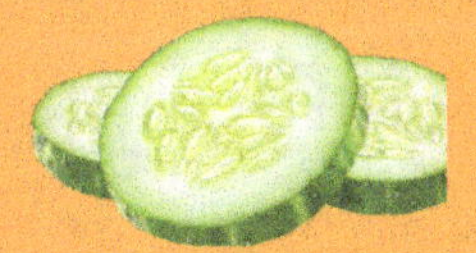

This Cookbook Belong to:

Name: _______________________

Copyright © 2024 by Vakare Rimkute

⚠ Disclaimer

The recipes and information presented in this cookbook are intended for general informational purposes only. While Vakare Rimkute has made every effort to ensure the accuracy and completeness of the content, they make no representations or warranties of any kind, express or implied, about the suitability or applicability of the recipes for any purpose .

Introduction to GERD

Welcome to the "GERD Diet Cookbook for Beginners," your essential guide to enjoying delicious meals while managing **gastroesophageal reflux disease** (**GERD**). This cookbook is designed for those new to the world of GERD-friendly eating, providing you with a variety of recipes that are both tasty and easy to prepare.

GERD can be challenging to manage, especially when it comes to meal planning. Many common ingredients and favorite dishes can trigger symptoms, making it difficult to enjoy eating. However, with the right knowledge and recipes, you can still savor flavorful meals that are gentle on your digestive system. In this cookbook, you will find a variety of recipes carefully curated to avoid common GERD triggers. From hearty breakfasts and satisfying lunches to delectable dinners and sweet treats, every recipe is crafted to be both tasty and GERD-friendly.

Each chapter focuses on a different type of meal, providing you with a comprehensive collection of dishes to choose from.

We also understand that managing GERD isn't just about the recipes you use; it's about making informed choices at the grocery store, in the kitchen, and even when dining out. That's why this cookbook includes helpful tips on what foods to avoid, what foods to include, and how to make substitutions to fit your dietary needs.

Our goal is to empower you with the knowledge and tools to take control of your diet and, ultimately, your health. With the "GERD Diet Cookbook for Beginners," you can transform your eating habits and enjoy meals that nourish your body without causing discomfort.

So, let's embark on this journey together. Turn the page to learn more about GERD and how you can manage it through diet, and then dive into the delicious recipes that await you. Happy cooking and eating!

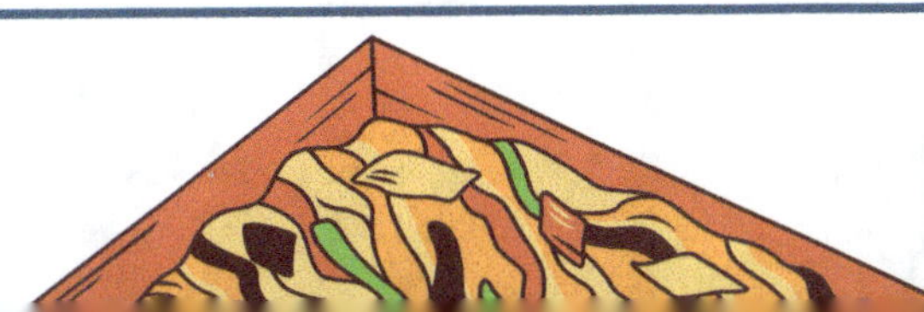

How to Use This Cookbook

- **Understand GERD and Diet:** Begin by reading the introductory sections on understanding GERD and the importance of diet in managing symptoms. This will provide you with the necessary background information.
- **Navigate by Meal Type**: The cookbook is organized into chapters based on meal types: Breakfasts, Snacks and Appetizers, Lunches, Dinners, Desserts, Beverages, Sauces and Dressings, and Side Dishes. Each chapter starts with an introduction to set the context.
- **Recipe Selection:** Each chapter contains 10 recipes. Browse through the chapters and select recipes that appeal to you. The recipes are crafted to be easy to follow, using ingredients that are less likely to trigger GERD symptoms.
- **Ingredient Substitutions:** If you have specific dietary needs or preferences, look for the substitution suggestions provided within the recipes. This will help you customize dishes while keeping them GERD-friendly.
- **Follow Dietary Tips:** Pay attention to the dietary tips provided, such as foods to avoid and foods to include. These tips are crucial for managing GERD effectively.
- **Plan Your Meals:** Use this cookbook to plan your meals throughout the day. Mix and match recipes from different chapters to create balanced, GERD-friendly meal plans.
- **Eating Out:** Refer to the tips on how to make GERD-friendly choices when dining out. These tips will help you maintain your diet even when you're away from home.

Table of Content

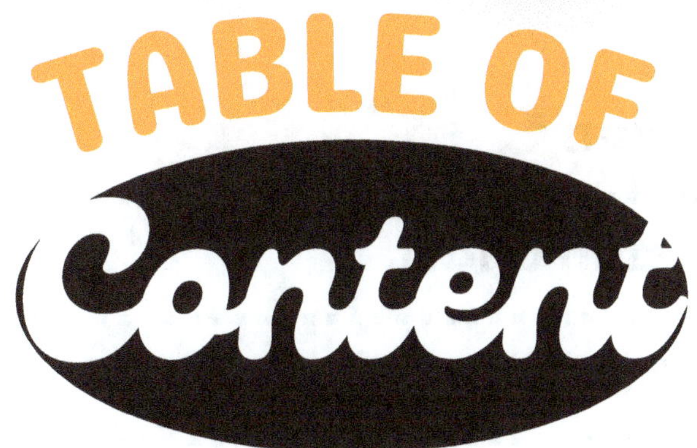

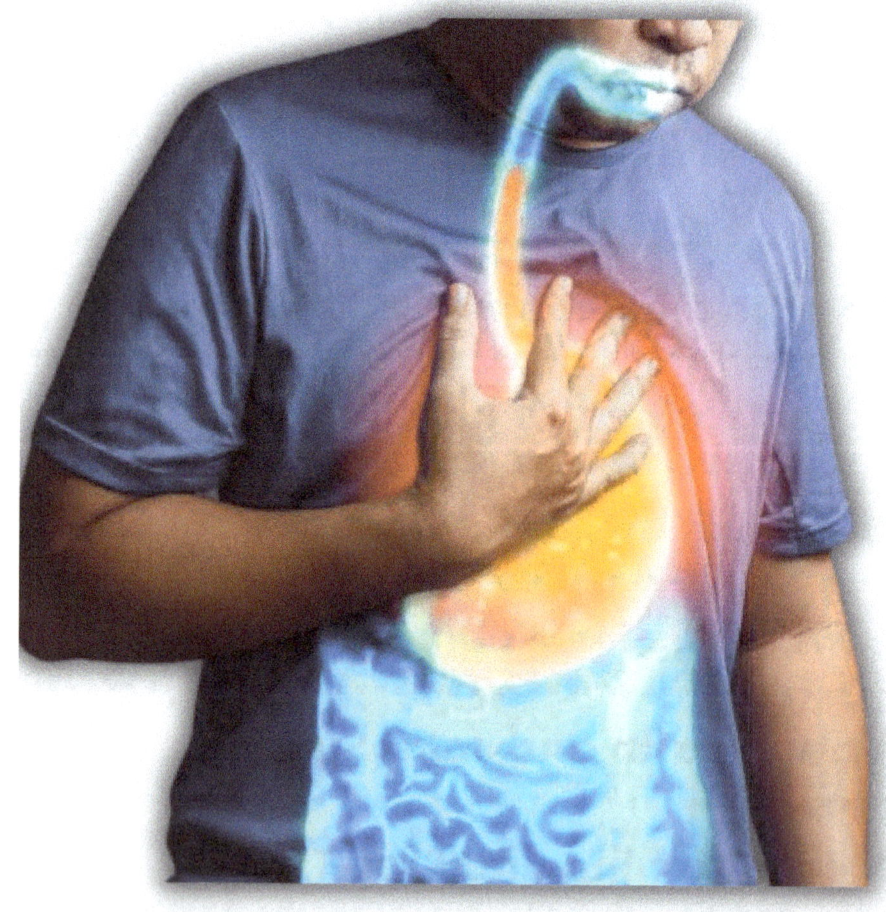

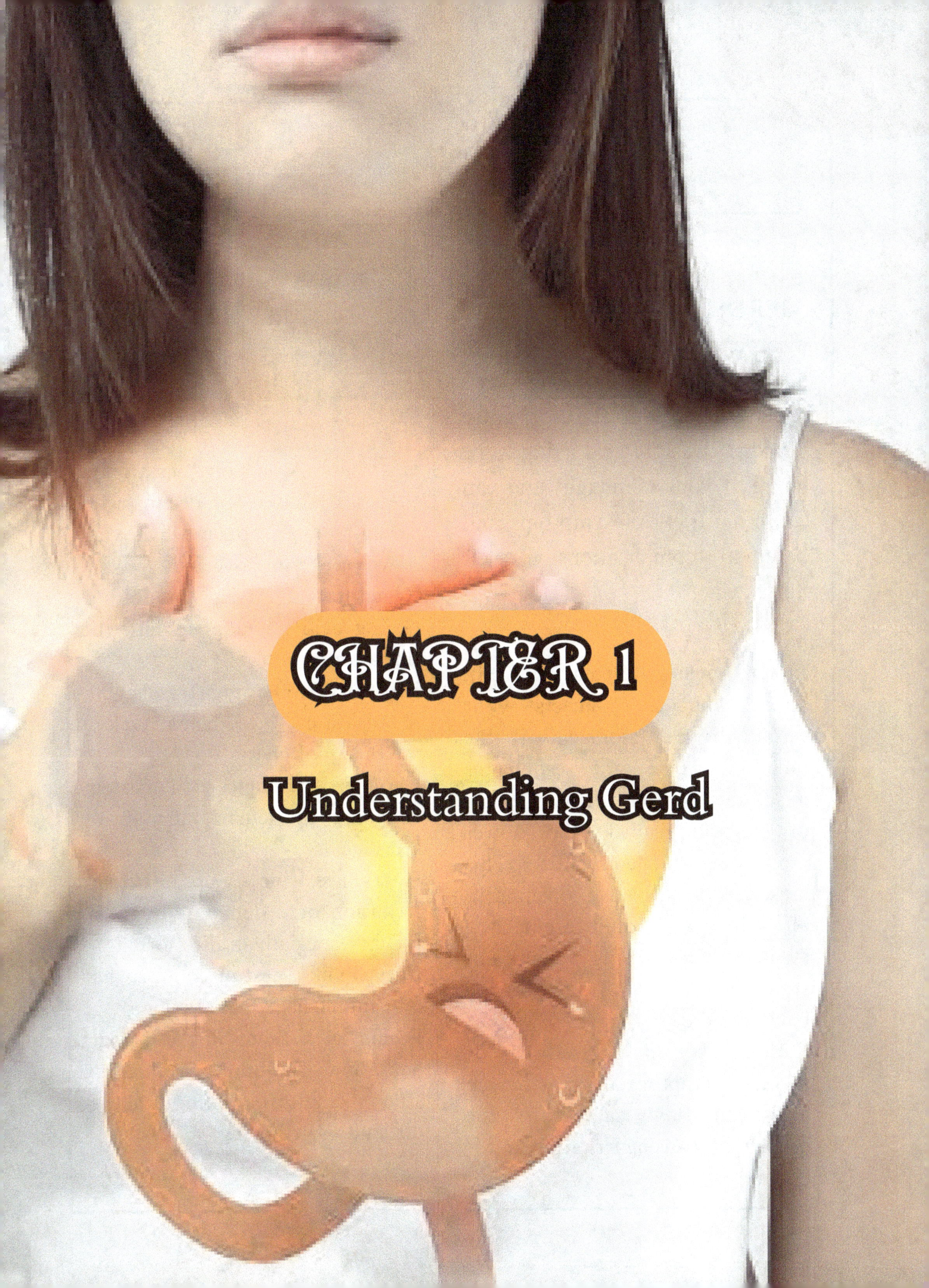

CHAPTER 1
Understanding Gerd

What is GERD?

Gastroesophageal Reflux Disease (GERD) is a chronic digestive disorder that occurs when stomach acid or, occasionally, bile flows back (refluxes) into the esophagus. This backwash of acid irritates the lining of your esophagus and can cause a variety of symptoms and potential complications if left untreated.

The Mechanics of GERD:

- **Lower Esophageal Sphincter (LES)**: The esophagus connects your throat to your stomach. At the junction where the esophagus meets the stomach, there is a ring of muscle called the lower esophageal sphincter (LES). This muscle acts as a valve, opening to allow food and liquid to enter the stomach and closing to prevent stomach contents from flowing back into the esophagus.
- **Reflux**: When the LES is weak or relaxes inappropriately, stomach acid can flow back into the esophagus, causing irritation and inflammation of the esophageal lining. This backward flow of acid is called reflux.

Symptoms of GERD

1. **Heartburn**: A burning sensation in the chest that often occurs after eating and can worsen when lying down or bending over.
2. **Regurgitation**: Sour or bitter-tasting acid backing up into the throat or mouth.
3. **Difficulty Swallowing (Dysphagia):** A sensation of food being stuck in the throat or chest.
4. **Chronic Cough**: Persistent coughing, particularly at night or after meals.
5. **Hoarseness or Sore Throat**: Irritation or inflammation of the throat, especially in the morning.
6. **Chest Pain**: Chest discomfort that may mimic heart pain (angina).
7. **Feeling of a Lump in the Throat**: Sensation of a lump or something stuck in the throat without actual difficulty swallowing.

Causes of GERD

GERD occurs when the lower esophageal sphincter (LES), a ring of muscle between the esophagus and stomach, becomes weak or relaxes inappropriately, allowing stomach acid and occasionally bile to flow back into the esophagus. The causes and contributing factors include:

1. Hiatal Hernia: A condition where part of the stomach pushes up through the diaphragm, weakening the LES.

2. Lifestyle factors:

- **Diet**: Consuming large meals, fatty or fried foods, spicy foods, chocolate, mint, garlic, onions, tomatoes, citrus fruits, and carbonated beverages can trigger GERD.
- **Smoking**: Tobacco use can weaken the LES and increase acid production.
- **Obesity**: Excess weight puts pressure on the abdomen and can push stomach contents into the esophagus.
- **Certain Medications**: Some medications, such as NSAIDs (non-steroidal anti-inflammatory drugs), calcium channel blockers, and certain asthma medications, can contribute to GERD symptoms.

3. Pregnancy: Hormonal changes and increased pressure on the abdomen during pregnancy can lead to GERD symptoms.

4. Delayed Stomach Emptying (Gastroparesis): Conditions that affect how well the stomach empties, such as diabetes, can increase the likelihood of reflux.

5. Age: GERD is more common in older adults due to changes in muscle tone and increased incidence of hiatal hernias.

Potential Complications:

- **Esophagitis**: Inflammation of the esophagus, which can lead to bleeding, ulcers, and chronic scarring.
- **Strictures**: Narrowing of the esophagus due to chronic inflammation and scarring, leading to swallowing difficulties.
- **Barrett's Esophagus:** A condition where the tissue lining the esophagus changes and can increase the risk of developing esophageal cancer.
- **Respiratory Problems**: Acid reflux can lead to chronic cough, laryngitis, asthma, and other respiratory issues.

Importance of Diet in Managing GERD

1. **Symptom Reduction:**
   - **Rationale**: Adhering to a GERD-friendly diet can significantly alleviate the hallmark symptoms of GERD, including heartburn, regurgitation, and chest pain.
   - **Implementation**: Avoid foods known to trigger GERD, such as fatty, spicy, and acidic foods, and instead opt for more suitable alternatives.

2. **Preventing Complications:**
   - **Rationale**: Chronic, unmanaged GERD can lead to serious health complications, such as esophagitis, esophageal strictures, Barrett's esophagus, and an increased risk of esophageal cancer.
   - **Implementation**: Following a GERD-friendly diet helps minimize acid reflux, thus protecting the esophagus from damage and reducing the risk of long-term complications

3. **Improving Digestive Health**:
   - **Rationale**: A balanced, GERD-friendly diet contributes to overall digestive health, preventing additional gastrointestinal issues and promoting efficient digestive function.
   - **Implementation**: Incorporate fiber-rich foods, lean proteins, and low-acid fruits and vegetables to support digestive health and prevent conditions like constipation.

4. **Enhancing Quality of Life:**
   - **Rationale**: Effective management of GERD symptoms through diet can lead to a significant improvement in daily comfort, sleep quality, and overall well-being.
   - **Implementation**: Adopt healthy eating habits such as consuming smaller, frequent meals, avoiding late-night eating, and choosing foods that do not trigger GERD symptoms to enhance daily comfort and energy levels.

5. **Supporting Weight Management:**
   - **Rationale**: Excess weight, particularly around the abdomen, can exacerbate GERD symptoms. A healthy diet aids in maintaining or achieving a healthy weight, thereby reducing GERD symptoms.
   - **Implementation**: Focus on nutrient-dense, low-calorie foods, and avoid high-fat, high-sugar items to support weight loss and reduce abdominal pressure, consequently decreasing reflux episodes.

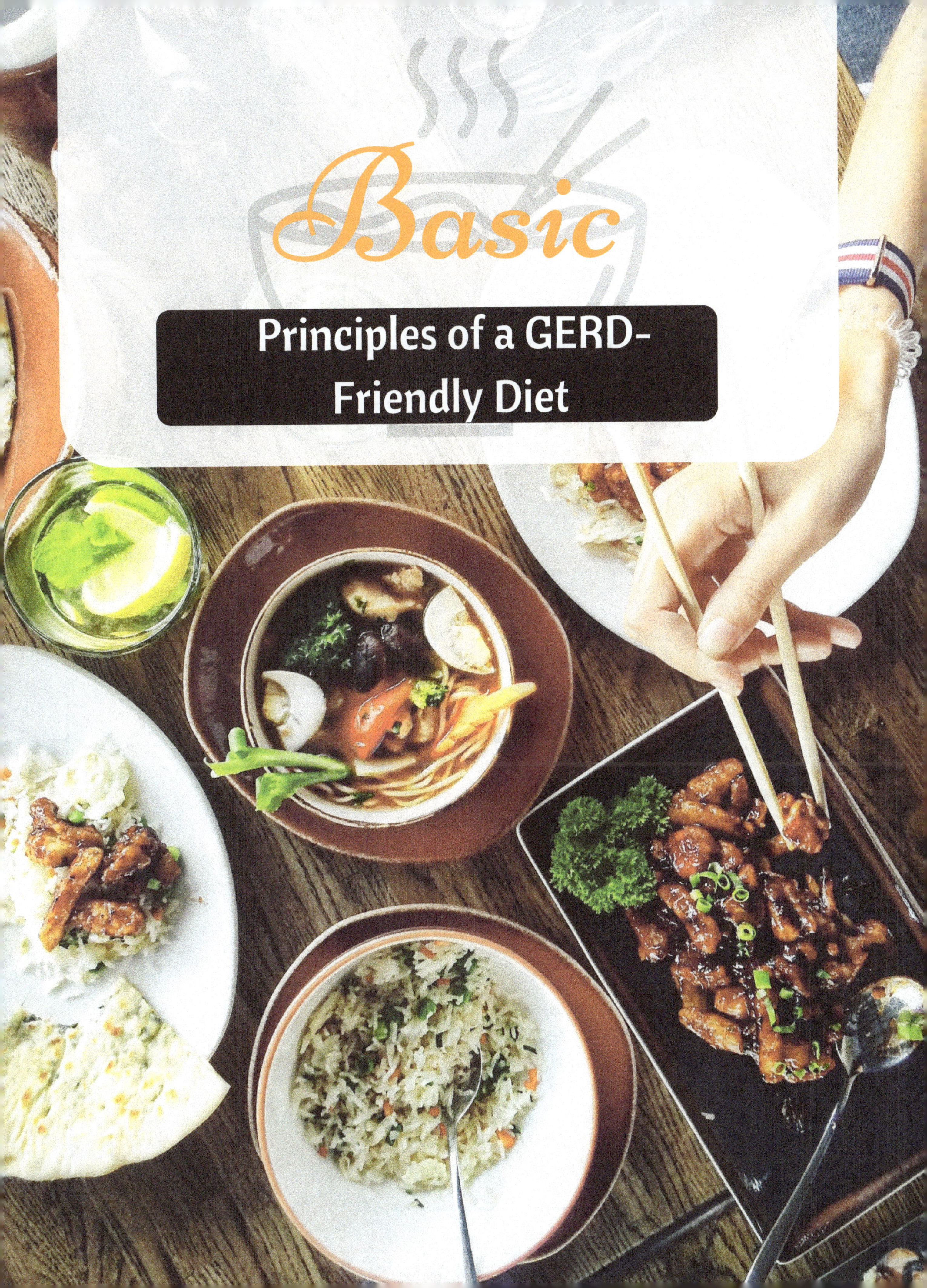
Basic
Principles of a GERD-Friendly Diet

Foods to Avoid

Fatty and Fried Foods

- **Impact**: These foods can slow down digestion and relax the lower esophageal sphincter (LES), increasing the risk of acid reflux.
- **Examples**: French fries, fried chicken, bacon, sausages, full-fat dairy products, and fatty cuts of meat.

Tomato-Based Products

- **Impact**: Tomatoes are acidic and can increase stomach acid, leading to reflux.
- **Examples**: Tomato sauce, ketchup, salsa, tomato soup, and raw tomatoes.

Spicy Foods

- **Impact**: Spicy foods can irritate the lining of the esophagus and increase stomach acid production, leading to heartburn.
- **Examples**: Hot peppers, chili powder, hot sauce, and dishes with heavy spices like curries.

Chocolate

- **Impact**: Chocolate contains caffeine and theobromine, which can relax the LES and increase the risk of acid reflux.
- **Examples**: Milk chocolate, dark chocolate, chocolate candy, and chocolate-flavored desserts.

Citrus Fruits and Juices

- **Impact**: Citrus fruits are highly acidic and can irritate the esophagus and worsen GERD symptoms.
- **Examples**: Oranges, lemons, limes, grapefruits, and their juices.

Caffeine

- **Impact**: Caffeine can relax the LES and increase stomach acid production.
- **Examples**: Coffee, tea, cola, and other caffeinated beverages.

Alcohol

- **Impact**: Alcohol can relax the LES, irritate the esophagus, and increase stomach acid production.
- **Examples**: Beer, wine, spirits, and mixed drinks containing alcohol.

Garlic and Onions

- **Impact**: Both garlic and onions can relax the LES and increase the likelihood of heartburn.
- **Examples**: Raw garlic, raw onions, garlic powder, and onion powder.

Carbonated Beverages

- **Impact**: Carbonated drinks can increase stomach pressure and cause belching, leading to acid reflux.
- **Examples**: Soda, sparkling water, and carbonated juices.

Mint and Mint-Flavored Products

- **Impact**: Mint can relax the LES, increasing the risk of acid reflux.
- **Examples**: Peppermint, spearmint, mint tea, and mint-flavored candies.

Foods to Include

Whole Grains

- **Examples**: Oatmeal, whole grain bread, brown rice, quinoa, barley
- **Benefits**: High in fiber, which aids digestion and can help prevent overeating.

Lean Proteins:

- **Examples**: Chicken breast, turkey, fish, tofu, legumes (beans, lentils)
- **Benefits**: Low-fat protein sources that don't exacerbate GERD symptoms.

Non-Citrus Fruits

- **Examples**: Bananas, melons, apples, pears
- **Benefits**: These fruits are less likely to trigger acid reflux compared to citrus fruits.

Low-Fat Dairy Products

- **Examples**: Skim milk, low-fat yogurt, low-fat cheese
- **Benefits**: Provides necessary nutrients without the high fat content that can trigger GERD.

Vegetables

- **Examples**: Leafy greens (spinach, kale), broccoli, carrots, green beans, zucchini
- **Benefits**: Low in fat and sugar, high in fiber and essential nutrients.

Healthy Fats

- **Examples**: Avocados, nuts (in moderation), seeds, olive oil
- **Benefits**: Healthy fats that are less likely to cause reflux symptoms.

Herbs and Mild Spices

- **Examples**: Basil, parsley, thyme, ginger
- **Benefits**: Adds flavor without the irritation that spicy foods can cause.

Root Vegetables

- **Examples**: Sweet potatoes, carrots, beets
- **Benefits**: Nutrient-dense and generally well-tolerated by people with GERD.

Non-Caffeinated Beverages

- **Examples**: Herbal teas (chamomile, ginger), water, non-citrus juices (apple, pear)
- **Benefits**: Helps stay hydrated without the acidity and caffeine that can trigger GERD.

Whole Grains

- **Examples**: Oatmeal, whole wheat pasta, quinoa
- **Benefits**: High in fiber, which helps with digestion and prevents overeating.

Egg Whites

- **Examples**: Scrambled egg whites, egg white omelets
- **Benefits**: High in protein, low in fat compared to whole eggs.

Melons

- **Examples**: Watermelon, cantaloupe, honeydew
- **Benefits**: Low-acid fruits that are less likely to cause reflux.

Basic Ingredients for a GERD-Friendly Diet

Whole Grains

- **Examples**: Oatmeal, whole grain bread, brown rice, quinoa, barley
- **Benefits**: High in fiber, which aids digestion and can help prevent overeating.

Lean Proteins:

- **Examples**: Chicken breast, turkey, fish, tofu, legumes (beans, lentils)
- **Benefits**: Low-fat protein sources that don't exacerbate GERD symptoms.

Non-Citrus Fruits

- **Examples**: Bananas, melons, apples, pears
- **Benefits**: These fruits are less likely to trigger acid reflux compared to citrus fruits.

Low-Fat Dairy Products

- **Examples**: Skim milk, low-fat yogurt, low-fat cheese
- **Benefits**: Provides necessary nutrients without the high fat content that can trigger GERD.

Vegetables

- **Examples**: Leafy greens (spinach, kale), broccoli, carrots, green beans, zucchini
- **Benefits**: Low in fat and sugar, high in fiber and essential nutrients.

Healthy Fats

- **Examples**: Avocados, nuts (in moderation), seeds, olive oil
- **Benefits**: Healthy fats that are less likely to cause reflux symptoms.

Herbs and Mild Spices

- **Examples**: Basil, parsley, thyme, ginger
- **Benefits**: Adds flavor without the irritation that spicy foods can cause.

Root Vegetables

- **Examples**: Sweet potatoes, carrots, beets
- **Benefits**: Nutrient-dense and generally well-tolerated by people with GERD.

Non-Caffeinated Beverages

- **Examples**: Herbal teas (chamomile, ginger), water, non-citrus juices (apple, pear)
- **Benefits**: Helps stay hydrated without the acidity and caffeine that can trigger GERD.

Whole Grains

- **Examples**: Oatmeal, whole wheat pasta, quinoa
- **Benefits**: High in fiber, which helps with digestion and prevents overeating.

Egg Whites

- **Examples**: Scrambled egg whites, egg white omelets
- **Benefits**: High in protein, low in fat compared to whole eggs.

Melons

- **Examples**: Watermelon, cantaloupe, honeydew
- **Benefits**: Low-acid fruits that are less likely to cause reflux.

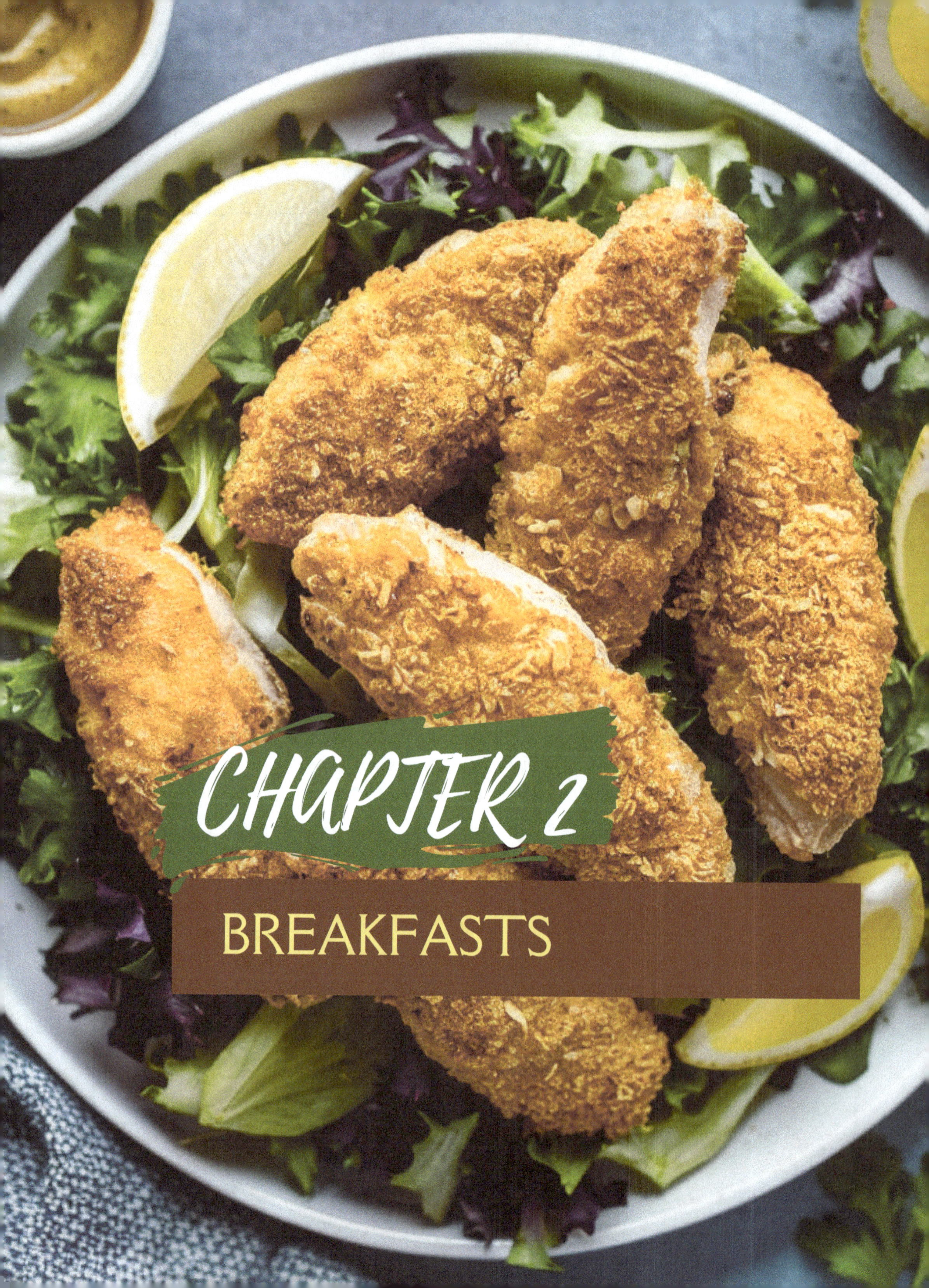
CHAPTER 2
BREAKFASTS

SPINACH AND MUSHROOM FRITTATA

Ingredients

- 1 cup fresh spinach, chopped
- 1 cup mushrooms, sliced
- 6 large eggs
- 1/4 cup milk (dairy or non-dairy)
- 1/2 cup shredded cheese (optional, can use dairy-free cheese)
- 1 small onion, finely chopped
- 1 clove garlic, minced
- Salt and pepper to taste
- 1 tablespoon olive oil

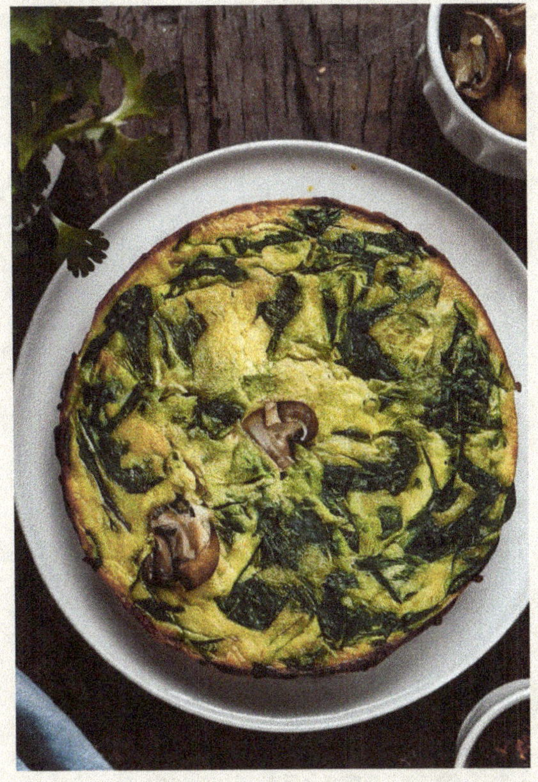

Instructions

- Preheat your oven to 375°F (190°C).
- In a large oven-safe skillet, heat the olive oil over medium heat.
- Add the chopped onion and garlic, sauté until fragrant and the onion is translucent, about 2-3 minutes.
- Add the sliced mushrooms to the skillet, cook until they release their moisture and start to brown, about 5 minutes.
- Add the chopped spinach to the skillet and cook until wilted, about 1-2 minutes.
- In a mixing bowl, whisk together the eggs, milk, salt, and pepper.
- Pour the egg mixture over the vegetables in the skillet. If using, sprinkle the shredded cheese evenly over the top.
- Cook on the stove for about 2-3 minutes until the edges start to set.
- Transfer the skillet to the preheated oven and bake for 10-12 minutes, or until the frittata is fully set and lightly golden on top.
- Remove from the oven, let it cool slightly, then slice into wedges and serve.

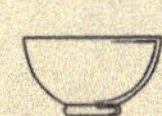 **Preparation Time : 10 min**

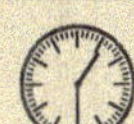 **Total Time : 25 min**

 **Servings : 4**

Nutritional Info

- Calories: 180
- Protein: 12g
- Fat: 12g
- Carbohydrates: 5g
- Fiber: 1g

SWEET POTATO AND KALE HASH

Ingredients

- 2 medium sweet potatoes, peeled and diced
- 1 bunch kale, stems removed and leaves chopped
- 1 onion, diced
- 2 garlic cloves, minced
- 1 tablespoon olive oil
- Salt and pepper, to taste

Instructions

- Heat olive oil in a large skillet over medium heat.
- Add onion and garlic, and sauté until onion is translucent.
- Add sweet potatoes and cook, stirring occasionally, until they start to soften, about 10 minutes.
- Stir in kale and cook until wilted.
- Season with salt and pepper.
- Serve hot.

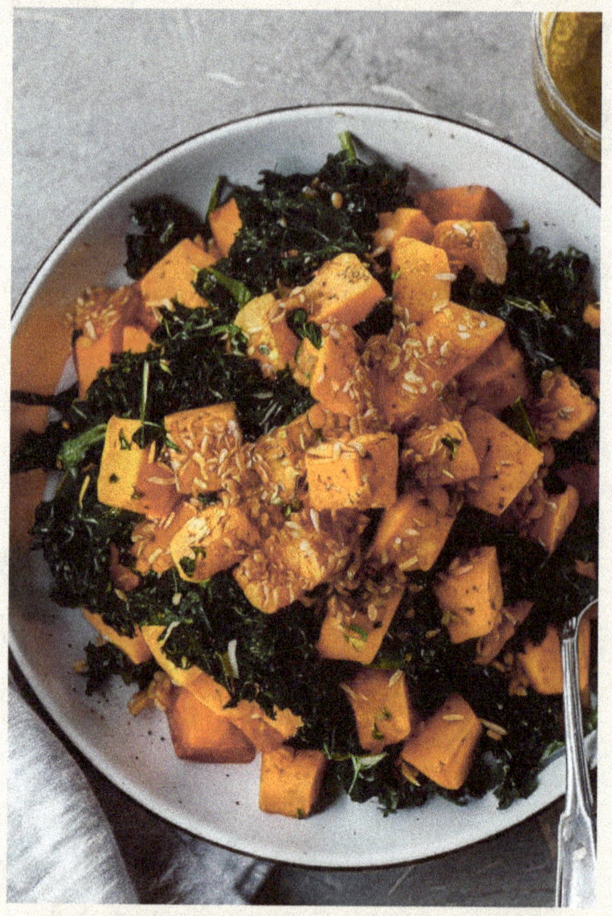

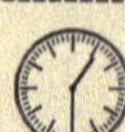
Preparation Time : 10 min

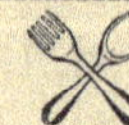
Total Time : 30 min

Servings : 4

Nutritional Info

- Calories: 180
- Fat: 4g
- Carbohydrates: 35g
- Fiber: 5g
- Protein: 3g

AVOCADO TOAST WITH POACHED EGG

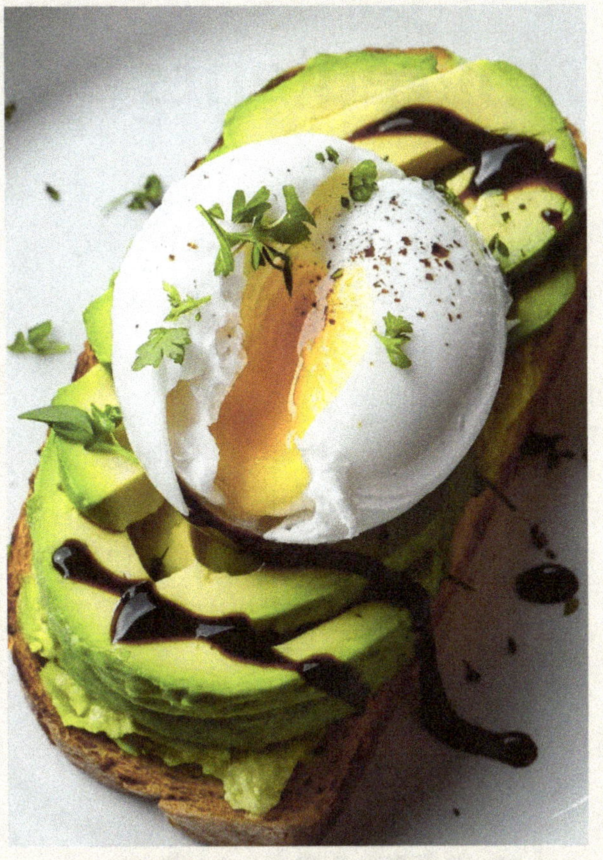

Ingredients

- 1 slice of whole grain bread
- 1/2 ripe avocado
- 1 egg
- Salt and pepper to taste
- Optional toppings: red pepper flakes, chopped chives.

Instructions

- Fill a small saucepan with water and bring it to a simmer.
- Crack the egg into a small bowl or cup.
- Create a gentle whirlpool in the water and carefully slide the egg into the center.
- Cook for about 3-4 minutes for a soft yolk, or longer for a firmer yolk.
- Remove the egg with a slotted spoon and place it on a paper towel to drain.
- While the egg is poaching, cut the avocado in half and remove the pit.
- Scoop out the flesh into a bowl and mash it with a fork.
- Toast the bread until golden brown and crispy.
- Spread the mashed avocado evenly onto the toasted bread.
- Place the poached egg on top.
- Season with additional salt and pepper if desired.
- Add any optional toppings like red pepper flakes, chopped chives, or a squeeze of lemon juice.
- Serve the avocado toast immediately and enjoy!

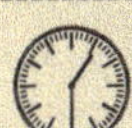 **Preparation Time : 5 min**

 **Total Time : 10 min**

Servings : 1

Nutritional Info

- Calories: 300 kcal
- Protein: 10g
- Fat: 20g
- Carbohydrates: 25g
- Fiber: 10g

TURMERIC AND GINGER SMOOTHIE

Ingredients

- 1 ripe banana
- 1 cup coconut milk (or any milk of your choice)
- 1/2 teaspoon ground turmeric
- 1/2 teaspoon grated ginger
- 1 tablespoon honey (optional, adjust to taste)
- Handful of ice cubes

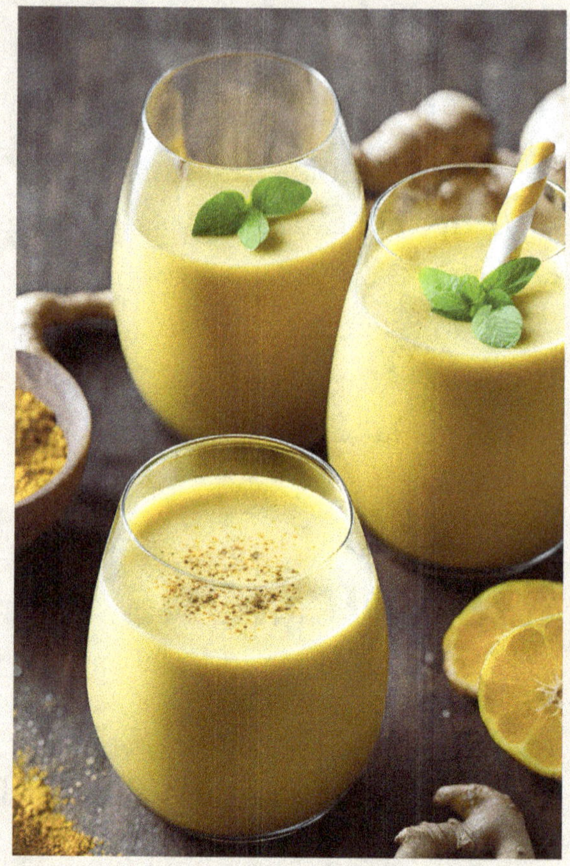

Instructions

- Peel and chop the banana.
- Add all ingredients to a blender.
- Blend until smooth and creamy.
- Taste and adjust sweetness if necessary by adding more honey.
- Serve immediately in glasses.

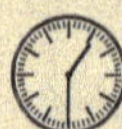 **Preparation Time : 5 min**

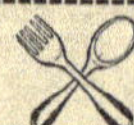 **Total Time : 5 min**

Servings : 2

Nutritional Info

- Calories: 120 kcal
- Fat: 6g
- Carbohydrates: 20g
- Protein: 1g
- Fiber: 3g

CHIA SEED BREAKFAST PUDDING

Ingredients

- 2 tablespoons chia seeds
- 1/2 cup almond milk (or any milk of your choice)
- 1/2 teaspoon vanilla extract
- 1 tablespoon honey or maple syrup (optional)
- Fresh fruits (such as berries, sliced banana, or mango) for topping
- Nuts or seeds for topping (such as sliced almonds, chopped walnuts, or pumpkin seeds)

Instructions

- In a bowl or jar, combine chia seeds, almond milk, vanilla extract, and honey or maple syrup (if using). Stir well to combine.
- Cover the bowl or jar and refrigerate overnight, or for at least 4 hours, to allow the chia seeds to absorb the liquid and thicken into a pudding-like consistency.
- Once the chia seed pudding has thickened, give it a good stir.
- Serve the chia seed pudding chilled, topped with your favorite fruits, nuts, or seeds.
- Enjoy your nutritious and delicious Chia Seed Breakfast Pudding!

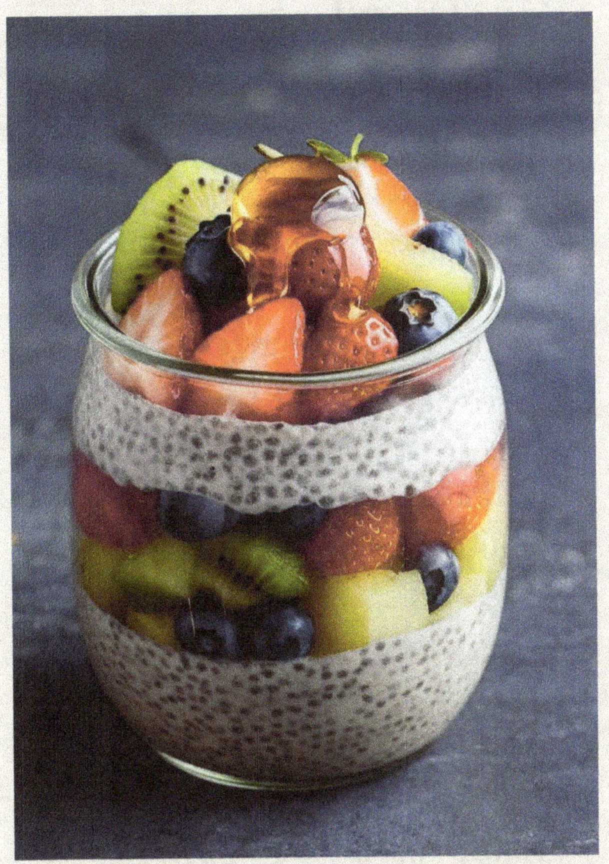

Preparation Time : 5 min

Total Time : 0 min

Servings : 1

Nutritional Info

- Calories: 220 kcal
- Protein: 6g
- Carbohydrates: 20g
- Fat: 14g
- Fiber: 10g

QUINOA AND BERRY BREAKFAST BOWL

Ingredients

- 1 cup quinoa
- 2 cups almond milk (or any milk of your choice)
- 1 tablespoon honey or maple syrup
- 1 teaspoon vanilla extract
- 1 cup mixed berries (strawberries, blueberries, raspberries)
- 1/4 cup chopped nuts (almonds, walnuts, or pecans)
- Optional toppings: sliced bananas, shredded coconut, chia seeds

Instructions

1. Rinse quinoa under cold water using a fine mesh strainer.
2. In a medium saucepan, combine quinoa and almond milk. Bring to a boil, then reduce heat to low and simmer for 15-20 minutes, or until quinoa is cooked and liquid is absorbed.
3. Remove from heat and stir in honey or maple syrup and vanilla extract.
4. Divide the cooked quinoa into serving bowls.
5. Top each bowl with mixed berries, chopped nuts, and any other desired toppings.
6. Serve warm or chilled.

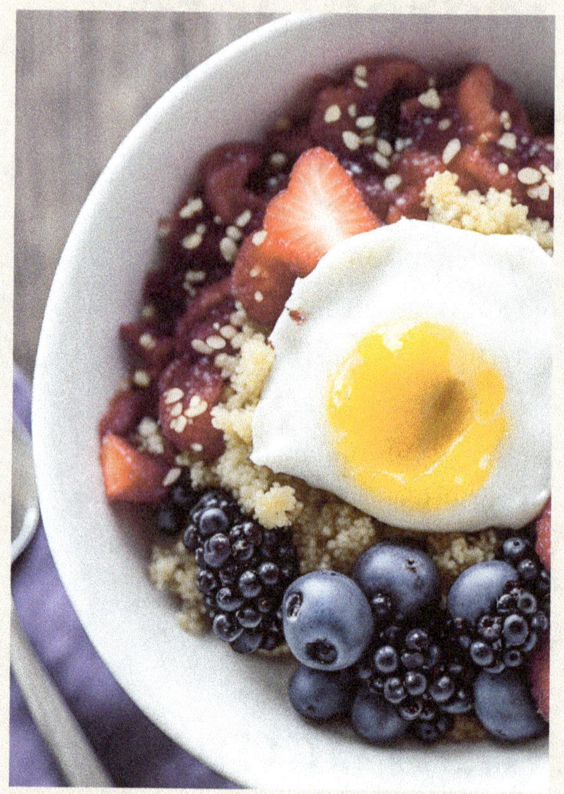

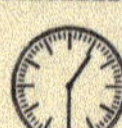 **Preparation Time : 5 min**

 **Total Time : 20 min**

Servings : 2

Nutritional Info

- Calories: 350 kcal
- Protein: 10g
- Carbohydrates: 55g
- Fat: 10g
- Fiber: 8g

BANANA OAT PANCAKES

Ingredients

- 1 ripe banana
- 1/2 cup rolled oats
- 2 eggs
- 1/2 teaspoon cinnamon
- 1/2 teaspoon vanilla extract
- Cooking spray or butter, for cooking
- Optional toppings: fresh berries, maple syrup, Greek yogurt

Instructions

- In a blender, combine the ripe banana, rolled oats, eggs, cinnamon, and vanilla extract. Blend until smooth.
- Heat a non-stick skillet or griddle over medium heat. Lightly coat with cooking spray or melt a small amount of butter.
- Pour the pancake batter onto the skillet, using about 1/4 cup for each pancake. Cook for 2-3 minutes, or until bubbles form on the surface.
- Flip the pancakes and cook for an additional 1-2 minutes, or until golden brown and cooked through.
- Remove the pancakes from the skillet and repeat with the remaining batter. Serve warm with your favorite toppings.

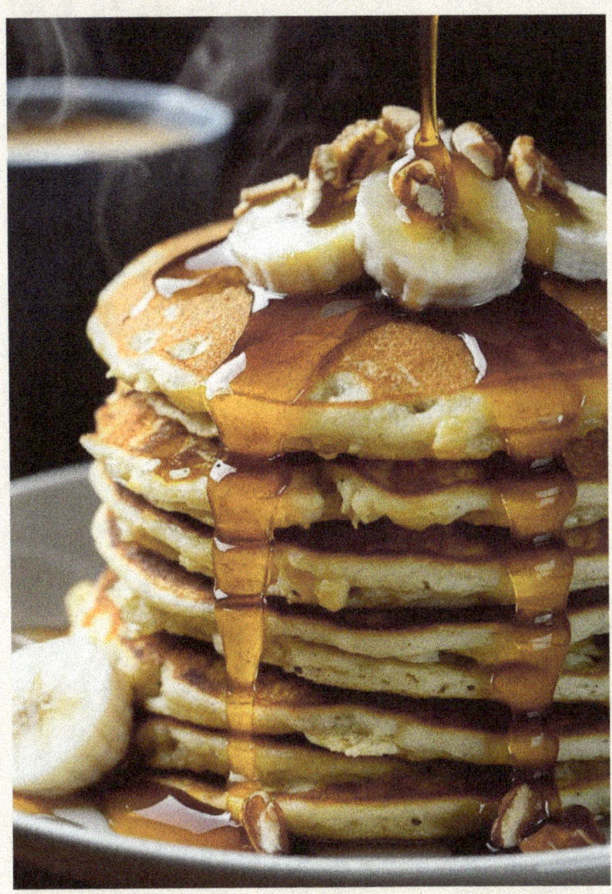

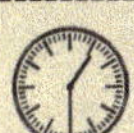
Preparation Time : 10 min

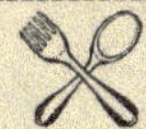
Total Time : 20 min

Servings : 2

Nutritional Info

- Calories: 250 kcal
- Protein: 10g
- Carbohydrates: 35g
- Fiber: 5g
- Sugars: 13g
- Fat: 8g

OATMEAL WITH FLAXSEEDS AND WALNUTS

Ingredients

- 1/2 cup rolled oats
- 1 cup water
- 1 tablespoon ground flaxseeds
- 2 tablespoons chopped walnuts
- Optional: honey or maple syrup for sweetness

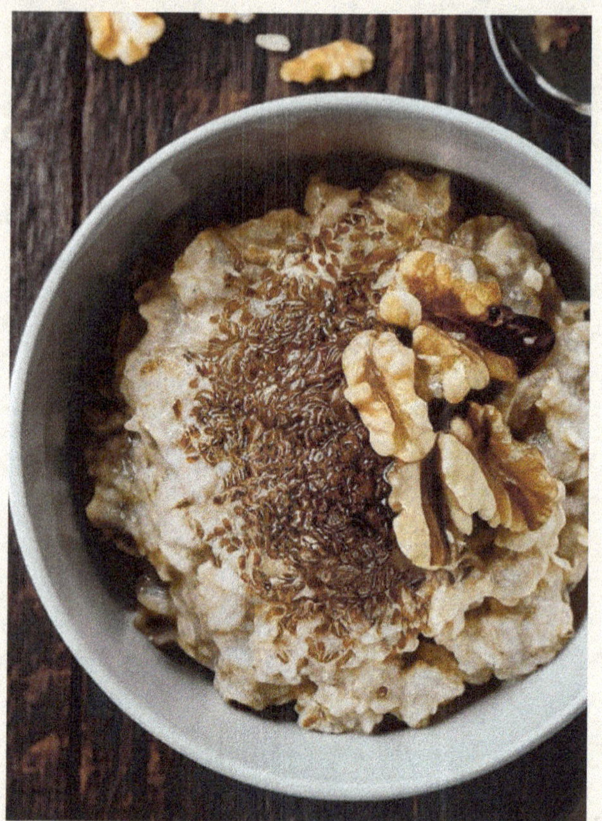

Instructions

- In a small saucepan, bring the water to a boil.
- Stir in the rolled oats and reduce heat to medium-low.
- Cook for about 5 minutes, stirring occasionally, until the oats are tender and creamy.
- Remove from heat and stir in the ground flaxseeds.
- Transfer the oatmeal to a serving bowl and sprinkle with chopped walnuts.
- Drizzle with honey or maple syrup if desired.
- Serve hot and enjoy!

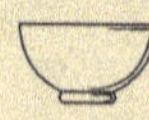 **Preparation Time : 2 min**

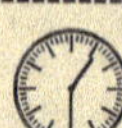 **Total Time : 7 min**

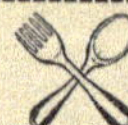 **Servings : 1**

Nutritional Info

- Calories: 270 kcal
- Protein: 9g
- Carbohydrates: 38g
- Fat: 11g
- Fiber: 7g

GREEK YOGURT PARFAIT WITH FRESH BERRIES

Ingredients

- 1 cup non-fat Greek yogurt
- 1/2 cup fresh strawberries, sliced
- 1/4 cup fresh blueberries
- 1/4 cup fresh raspberries
- 1 tablespoon honey (optional)
- 1/4 cup granola (optional for added texture)

Instructions

- Wash and slice the strawberries.
- Wash the blueberries and raspberries.
- In a glass or bowl, start by adding a layer of Greek yogurt at the bottom.
- Add a layer of sliced strawberries, blueberries, and raspberries on top of the yogurt.
- Drizzle a small amount of honey over the berries if using.
- Add another layer of Greek yogurt on top of the berries.
- Repeat the layers until all ingredients are used, finishing with berries on top.
- Sprinkle granola on top for added texture and crunch, if desired.
- Serve immediately or refrigerate for up to 1 hour to allow flavors to meld.

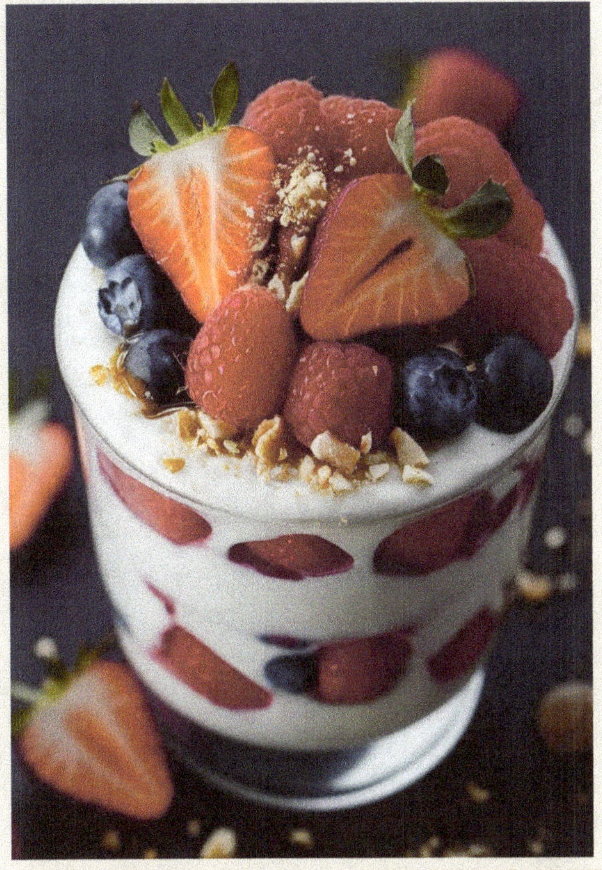

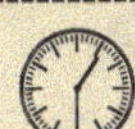 **Preparation Time : 10 min**

 **Total Time : 10 min**

Servings : 1

Nutritional Info

Calories: 150
Protein: 15g
Carbohydrates: 20g
Fat: 2g
Fiber: 4g

GREEN DETOX SMOOTHIE

Ingredients

- 1 cup spinach leaves
- 1/2 cucumber, peeled and chopped
- 1/2 green apple, cored and chopped
- 1/2 lemon, juiced
- 1/2 inch fresh ginger, peeled
- 1/2 cup coconut water or plain water
- Ice cubes (optional)

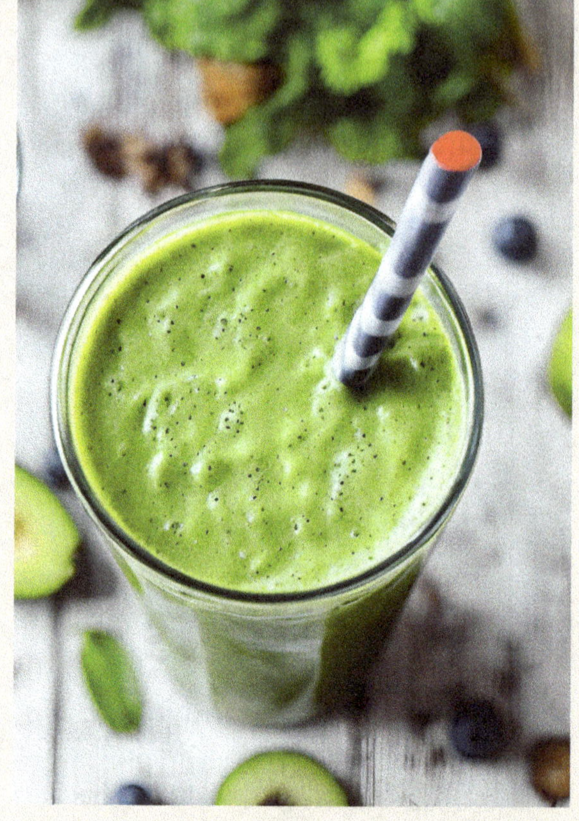

Instructions

- Place all ingredients in a blender.
- Blend until smooth and creamy.
- Add more water if needed to reach desired consistency.
- Pour into a glass and serve immediately.

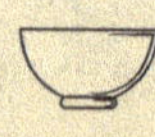 **Preparation Time : 5 min**

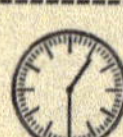 **Total Time : 5 min**

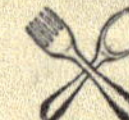 **Servings : 1**

Nutritional Info

- Calories: 70
- Protein: 2g
- Carbohydrates: 16g
- Fiber: 4g
- Fat: 0.5g

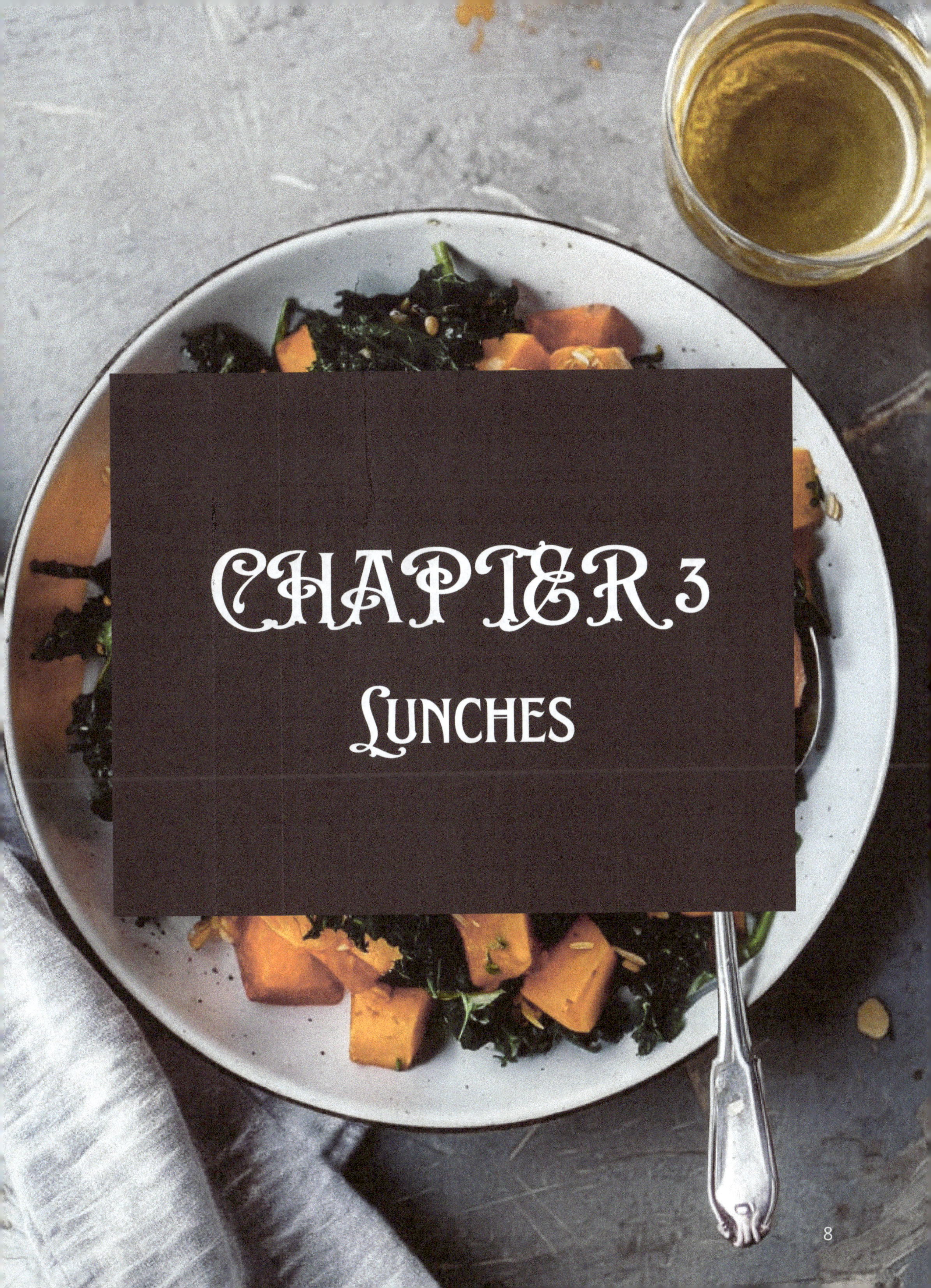

CHAPTER 3
Lunches

SPINACH AND STRAWBERRY SALAD

Ingredients

- 6 cups fresh baby spinach leaves
- 1 pint strawberries, hulled and sliced
- 1/4 cup sliced almonds
- 1/4 cup crumbled feta cheese
- Balsamic vinaigrette dressing

Instructions

- Wash the spinach leaves thoroughly and pat them dry with paper towels or a clean kitchen towel.
- In a large salad bowl, combine the spinach leaves, sliced strawberries, sliced almonds, and crumbled feta cheese.
- Drizzle the desired amount of balsamic vinaigrette dressing over the salad. Toss gently to coat all the ingredients evenly.
- Serve immediately as a refreshing side salad or light meal.

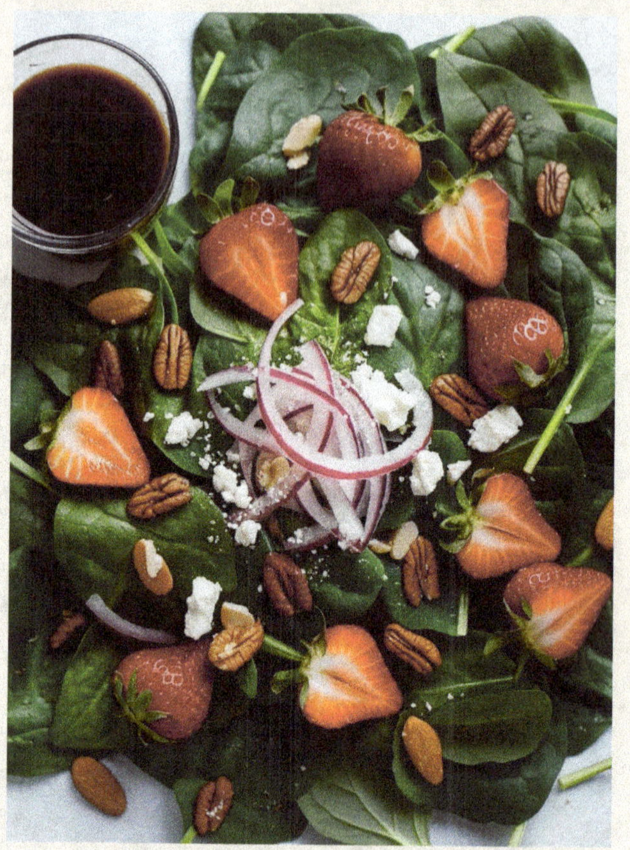

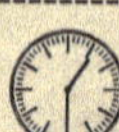 **Preparation Time : 10 min**

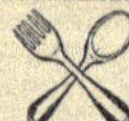 **Total Time : 10 min**

Servings : 4

Nutritional Info

- Calories: 120
- Total Fat: 7g
- Saturated Fat: 1.5g
- Cholesterol: 5mg
- Sodium: 140mg
- Dietary Fiber: 4g

GRILLED CHICKEN AND VEGETABLE SALAD

Ingredients

- 2 boneless, skinless chicken breasts
- 2 tablespoons olive oil
- 1 teaspoon garlic powder
- Salt and pepper to taste
- 4 cups mixed salad greens
- 1 bell pepper, sliced
- 1 cup cherry tomatoes, halved
- 1 small red onion, thinly sliced
- 1/4 cup balsamic vinaigrette dressing

Instructions

- Preheat your grill to medium-high heat.
- In a small bowl, mix together olive oil, garlic powder, salt, and pepper. Brush this mixture onto both sides of the chicken breasts.
- Grill the chicken breasts for about 6-8 minutes per side, or until cooked through and no longer pink in the center. Remove from the grill and let them rest for a few minutes before slicing.
- While the chicken is cooking, prepare the vegetables. In a large bowl, toss together the mixed salad greens, bell pepper slices, cherry tomatoes, and red onion slices.
- Once the chicken has rested, slice it thinly.
- Arrange the grilled chicken slices on top of the salad vegetables.
- Drizzle the balsamic vinaigrette dressing over the salad.
- Serve immediately and enjoy!

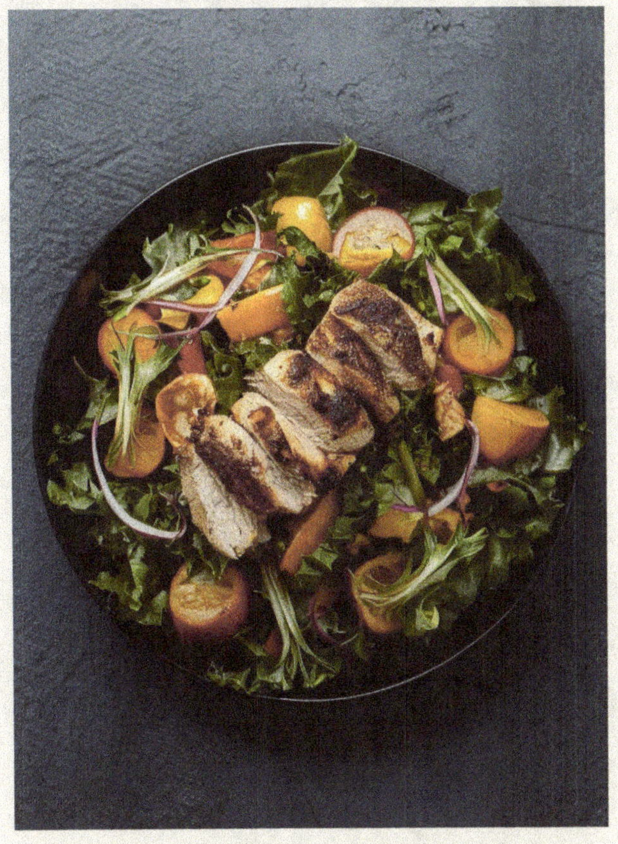

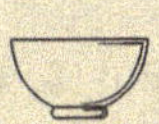 **Preparation Time : 15 min**

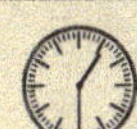 **Total Time : 30 min**

 **Servings : 4**

Nutritional Info

- Calories: 250 kcal
- Protein: 25g
- Carbohydrates: 15g
- Fat: 10g
- Fiber: 5g

AVOCADO AND BLACK BEAN WRAP

Ingredients

- 1 can (15 oz) black beans, drained and rinsed
- 1 ripe avocado, diced
- 1 cup cherry tomatoes, halved
- 1/4 cup red onion, finely chopped
- 1/4 cup fresh cilantro, chopped
- Juice of 1 lime
- Salt and pepper to taste
- 4 whole wheat tortillas
- 1/2 cup shredded lettuce (optional)

Instructions

- In a medium bowl, combine black beans, avocado, cherry tomatoes, red onion, cilantro, lime juice, salt, and pepper. Gently toss to mix all ingredients well.
- Lay the tortillas flat on a clean surface. Divide the black bean and avocado mixture evenly among the tortillas, placing it in the center of each.
- If using, sprinkle shredded lettuce over the mixture.
- Fold the sides of the tortillas over the filling, then roll them up tightly.
- Serve immediately, or wrap in foil or parchment paper to take on the go.

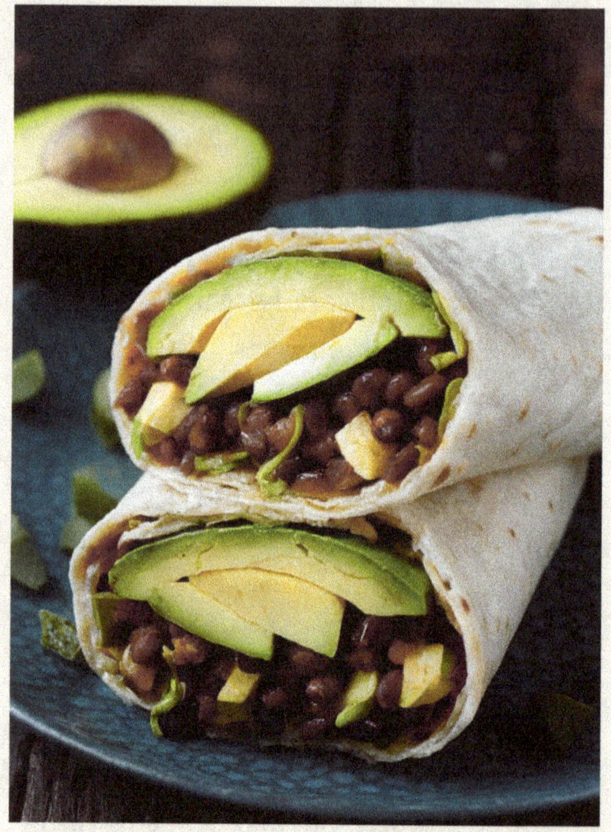

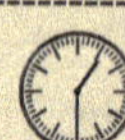 **Preparation Time : 10 min**

 **Total Time : 10 min**

Servings : 4

Nutritional Info

- Calories: 290
- Protein: 10g
- Fat: 10g
- Carbohydrates: 40g
- Fiber: 12g

ROASTED BEET AND GOAT CHEESE SALAD

Ingredients

- 4 medium beets, washed and trimmed
- 2 tablespoons olive oil
- Salt and pepper to taste
- 4 cups mixed greens (e.g., arugula, spinach, and kale)
- 1/2 cup crumbled goat cheese
- 1/4 cup chopped walnuts
- 1/4 cup balsamic vinaigrette

Instructions

- Preheat your oven to 400°F (200°C).
- Wrap each beet in aluminum foil and place them on a baking sheet.
- Roast for 45 minutes or until tender when pierced with a fork.
- Remove from the oven and let cool.
- Once cooled, peel the beets and cut them into wedges.
- In a large bowl, toss the mixed greens with olive oil, salt, and pepper.
- Add the roasted beet wedges, crumbled goat cheese, and chopped walnuts.
- Drizzle the balsamic vinaigrette over the salad and gently toss to combine.
- Divide the salad among four plates and serve immediately.

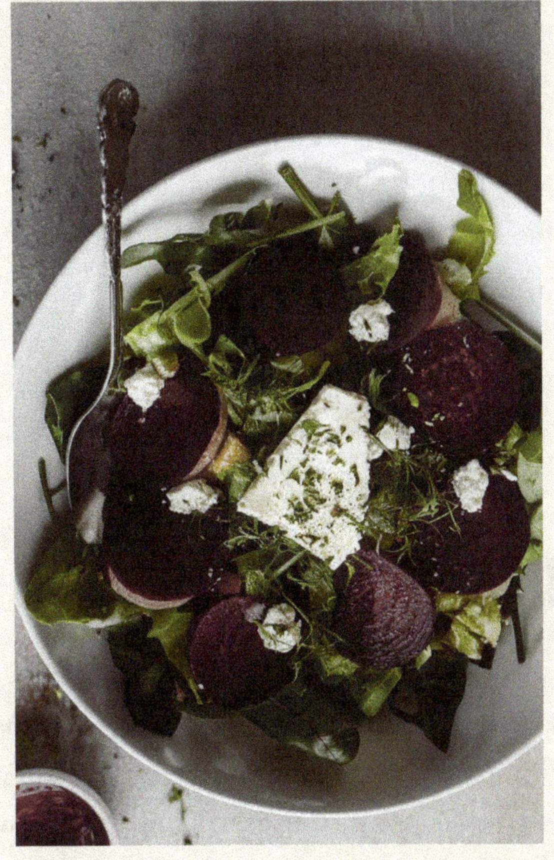

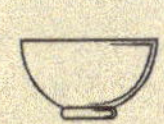 **Preparation Time : 15 min**

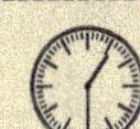 **Total Time : 60 min**

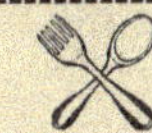 **Servings : 4**

Nutritional Info

- Calories: 210
- Protein: 6g
- Carbohydrates: 18g
- Fat: 14g
- Fiber: 4g

SALMON AND ASPARAGUS SALAD

Ingredients

- 2 salmon fillets
- 1 bunch of asparagus, trimmed
- 2 tablespoons olive oil
- Salt and pepper to taste
- 4 cups mixed salad greens
- 1 avocado, sliced
- 1/4 cup cherry tomatoes, halved
- 2 tablespoons balsamic vinegar

Instructions

- Preheat oven to 400°F (200°C).
- Place salmon fillets on a baking sheet lined with parchment paper. Drizzle with 1 tablespoon of olive oil and season with salt and pepper. Bake for 12-15 minutes until salmon is cooked through.
- While the salmon is baking, toss asparagus spears with the remaining olive oil, salt, and pepper. Roast in the oven for 8-10 minutes until tender but still crisp.
- In a large bowl, combine mixed salad greens, avocado slices, and cherry tomatoes.
- Once the salmon and asparagus are cooked, let them cool slightly. Then, flake the salmon into chunks and add it to the salad along with the asparagus.
- Drizzle balsamic vinegar over the salad and gently toss to combine.
- Serve immediately.

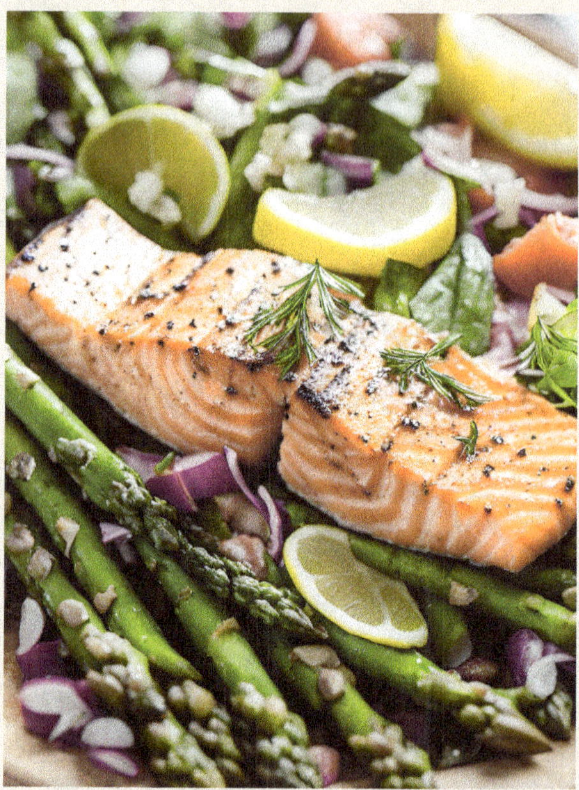

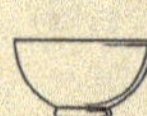 **Preparation Time : 10 min**

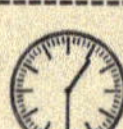 **Total Time : 25 min**

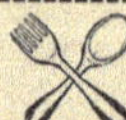 **Servings : 2**

Nutritional Info

- Calories: 450 kcal
- Protein: 28g
- Carbohydrates: 15g
- Fat: 33g
- Fiber: 9g

SWEET POTATO AND LENTIL STEW

Ingredients

- 1 tablespoon olive oil
- 1 onion, chopped
- 2 cloves garlic, minced
- 2 medium sweet potatoes, peeled and diced
- 1 cup dried green lentils, rinsed
- 4 cups vegetable broth
- 1 can (14 ounces) diced tomatoes
- 1 teaspoon ground cumin
- 1 teaspoon ground coriander
- Salt and pepper to taste

Instructions

- In a large pot or Dutch oven, heat the olive oil over medium heat.
- Add the chopped onion and minced garlic. Sauté until the onion is translucent, about 3-4 minutes.
- Add the diced sweet potatoes and rinsed lentils to the pot.
- Pour in the vegetable broth and diced tomatoes. Stir to combine.
- Season the stew with ground cumin, ground coriander, salt, and pepper.
- Bring the stew to a simmer, then reduce the heat to low. Cover and cook for 25-30 minutes, or until the sweet potatoes and lentils are tender.
- Taste and adjust seasoning if needed.
- Serve the stew hot, garnished with fresh cilantro or parsley if desired.

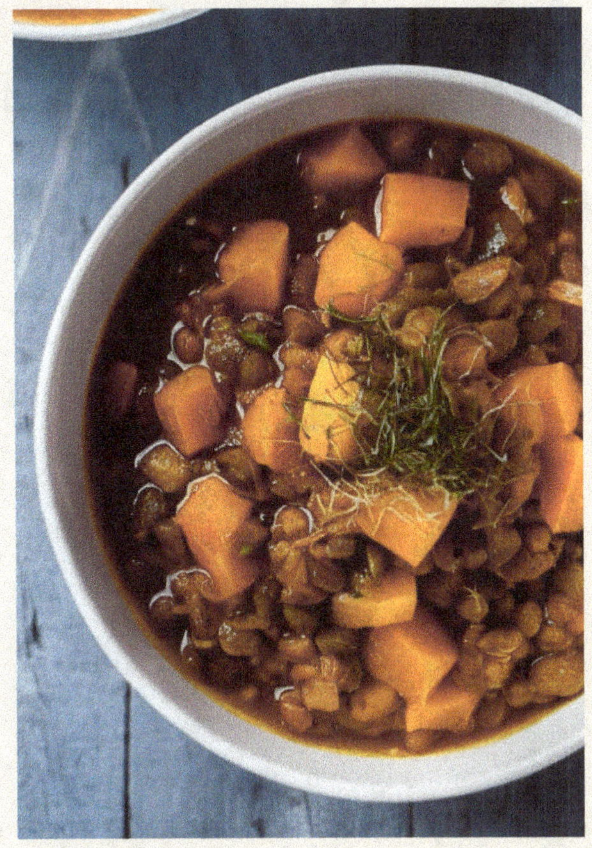

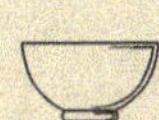 **Preparation Time : 10 min**

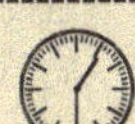 **Total Time : 40 min**

 **Servings : 4**

Nutritional Info

- Calories: 315 kcal
- Protein: 13g
- Carbohydrates: 58g
- Fat: 4g
- Fiber: 15g

TOFU AND BROCCOLI STIR-FRY

Ingredients

- 1 block firm tofu, drained and cubed
- 2 cups broccoli florets
- 2 tablespoons soy sauce (or tamari for gluten-free)
- 1 tablespoon sesame oil
- 2 cloves garlic, minced
- 1 tablespoon grated ginger
- 2 tablespoons olive oil (for cooking)

Instructions

- Heat olive oil in a large skillet or wok over medium-high heat.
- Add cubed tofu to the skillet and cook until golden brown on all sides, about 5-7 minutes. Remove tofu from skillet and set aside.
- In the same skillet, add broccoli florets and cook for 3-4 minutes until they are bright green and slightly tender.
- Add minced garlic and grated ginger to the skillet, stirring constantly for about 1 minute until fragrant.
- Return the cooked tofu to the skillet and pour soy sauce and sesame oil over the tofu and broccoli mixture. Stir well to coat everything evenly.
- Cook for an additional 2-3 minutes until the sauce has thickened slightly and everything is heated through.
- Remove from heat and garnish with sesame seeds and sliced green onions if desired.
- Serve hot over cooked rice or quinoa.

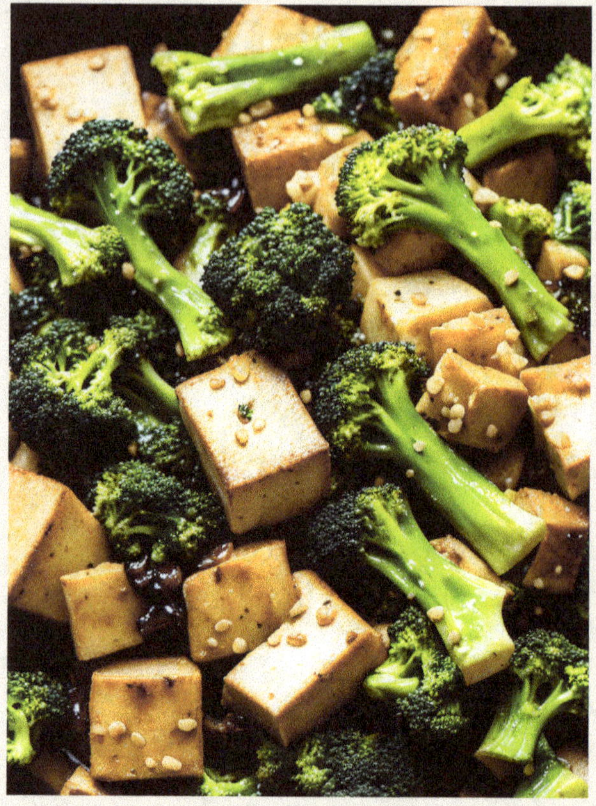

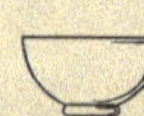 **Preparation Time : 10min**

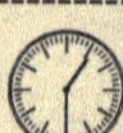 **Total Time : 20 min**

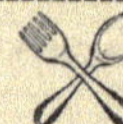 **Servings : 2**

Nutritional Info

- Calories: 250 kcal
- Protein: 15g
- Carbohydrates: 10g
- Fat: 18g
- Fiber: 5g

SPICY TUNA AND AVOCADO BOWL

Ingredients

- 1 can (5 oz) of tuna in water, drained
- 1 ripe avocado, diced
- 1 cup cooked brown rice (optional, adjust points if included)
- 1 cup mixed greens
- 1/2 cup shredded carrots
- 1/2 cup sliced cucumber
- 1/4 cup chopped green onions
- 1 tbsp soy sauce (low sodium)
- 1 tsp sesame oil
- 1 tsp Sriracha (adjust to taste)
- 1 tbsp lime juice
- 1 tbsp sesame seeds

Instructions

- Prepare the Ingredients: Drain the tuna and place it in a medium bowl. Dice the avocado and set aside. Cook the brown rice if using.
- Make the Dressing: In a small bowl, whisk together the soy sauce, sesame oil, Sriracha, and lime juice.
- Combine Ingredients: In the bowl with the tuna, add the mixed greens, shredded carrots, sliced cucumber, chopped green onions, and diced avocado. Pour the dressing over the mixture.
- Mix Well: Gently toss all the ingredients together until evenly coated with the dressing.
- Serve: Divide the mixture into bowls, sprinkle with sesame seeds, and season with salt and pepper to taste. Serve immediately.
- Optional: Serve over a bed of cooked brown rice for a heartier meal.

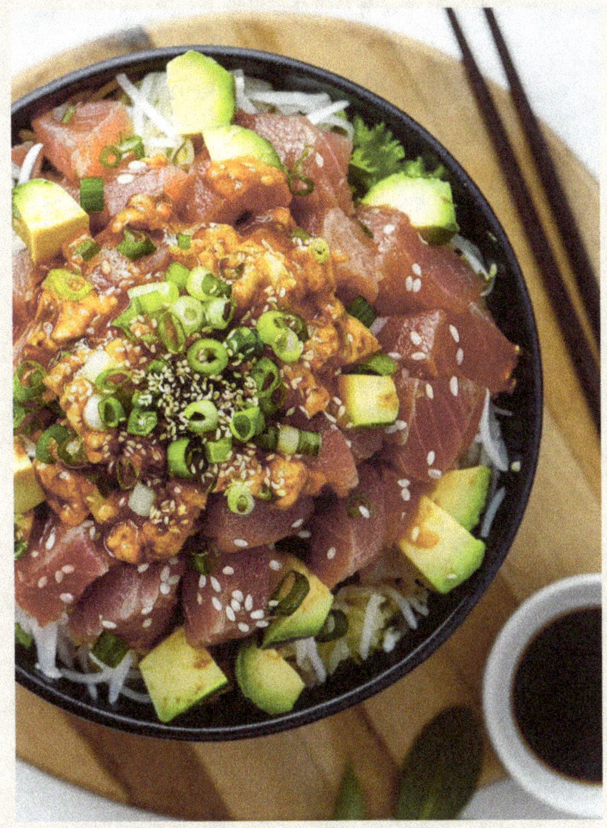

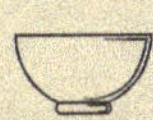 **Preparation Time : 10 min**

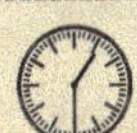 **Total Time : 10 min**

 **Servings : 1**

Nutritional Info

- Calories: 320 (without brown rice)
- Protein: 20g
- Carbohydrates: 14g
- Fat: 22g
- Fiber: 8g

CHICKEN CAESAR SALAD

Ingredients

- 2 boneless, skinless chicken breasts
- 1 tablespoon olive oil
- 1 teaspoon garlic powder
- Salt and pepper to taste
- 1 large head of romaine lettuce, chopped
- 1/2 cup cherry tomatoes, halved
- 1/4 cup grated Parmesan cheese
- 1/2 cup croutons (optional)
- Lemon wedges for garnish

Instructions

- Preheat your oven to 375°F (190°C).
- Rub the chicken breasts with olive oil, garlic powder, salt, and pepper.
- Place the chicken breasts on a baking sheet and bake for 20 minutes, or until the internal temperature reaches 165°F (74°C).
- Allow the chicken to rest for 5 minutes before slicing.
- While the chicken is baking, chop the romaine lettuce and place it in a large salad bowl.
- Add the halved cherry tomatoes and grated Parmesan cheese to the bowl.
- If using croutons, add them to the salad as well.
- Once the chicken has rested, slice it into thin strips.
- Arrange the sliced chicken on top of the salad.
- Serve the salad with lemon wedges on the side for squeezing over the top.
- Divide the salad into four servings.
- Enjoy your Chicken Caesar Salad without dressing, optionally squeezing fresh lemon juice over the top for extra flavor.

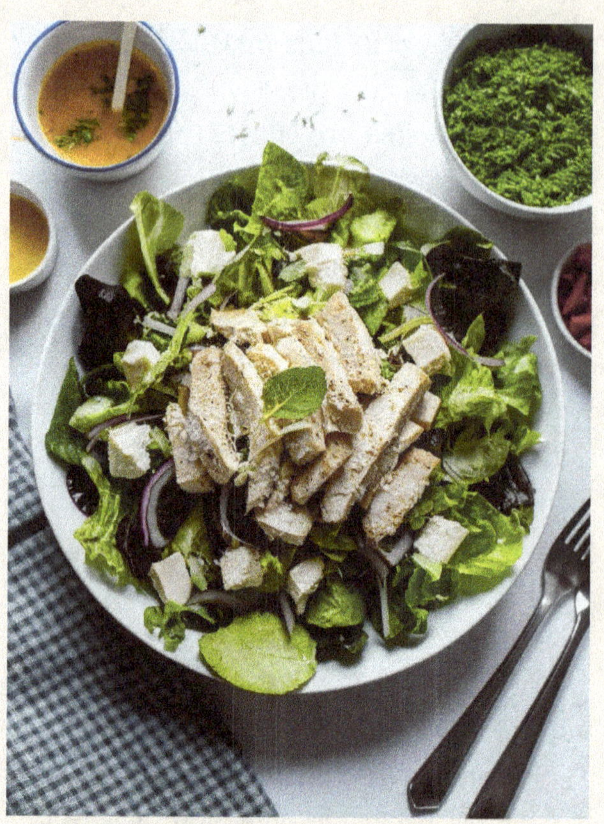

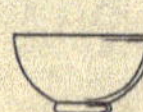 **Preparation Time : 15 min**

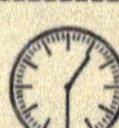 **Total Time : 35 min**

 **Servings : 4**

Nutritional Info

- Calories: 220
- Protein: 30g
- Carbohydrates: 8g
- Fat: 8g
- Fiber: 2g

MEDITERRANEAN CHICKPEA BOWL

Ingredients

- 1 can (15 oz) chickpeas, drained and rinsed
- 1 cup cherry tomatoes, halved
- 1 cucumber, diced
- 1/2 red onion, thinly sliced
- 1/4 cup Kalamata olives, pitted and sliced
- 2 tablespoons extra virgin olive oil
- 1 tablespoon lemon juice
- 1 teaspoon dried oregano
- Salt and pepper to taste

Instructions

- In a large bowl, combine the chickpeas, cherry tomatoes, cucumber, red onion, and Kalamata olives.
- In a small bowl, whisk together the extra virgin olive oil, lemon juice, dried oregano, salt, and pepper.
- Pour the dressing over the chickpea mixture and toss until well combined.
- Divide the chickpea mixture into serving bowls.
- Top with crumbled feta cheese and fresh parsley if desired.
- Serve immediately and enjoy!

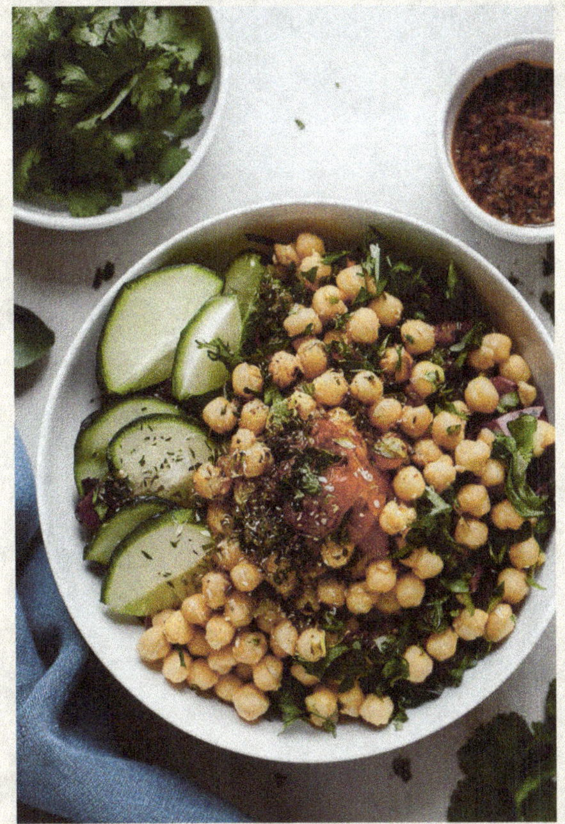

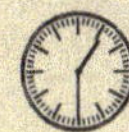 **Preparation Time : 10 min**

 **Total Time : 10 min**

Servings : 2

Nutritional Info

- Calories: 320 kcal
- Total Fat: 18g
- Saturated Fat: 2.5g
- Trans Fat: 0g
- Cholesterol: 0mg

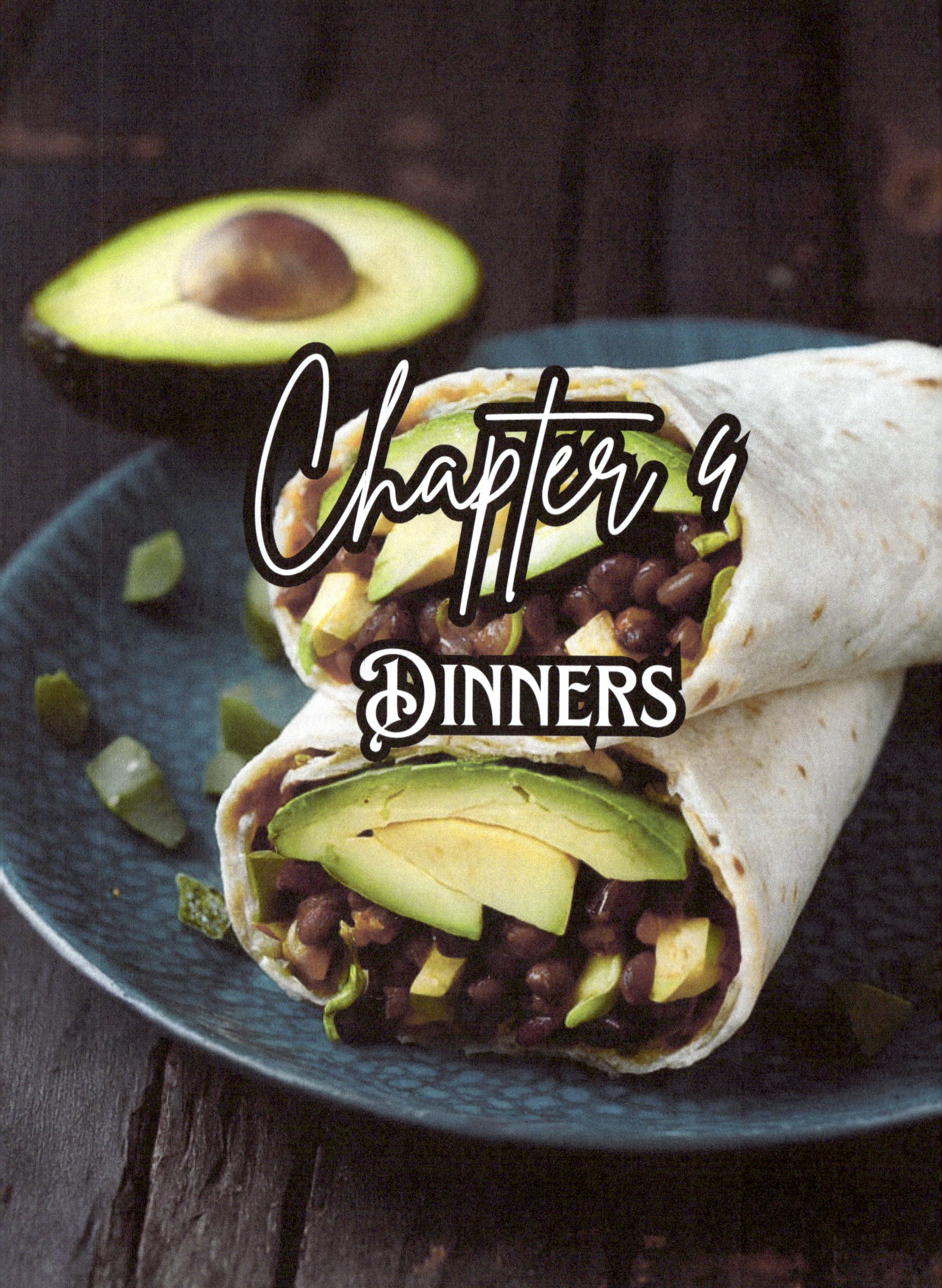
Chapter 4
DINNERS

BAKED SALMON WITH LEMON AND DILL

Ingredients

- 4 salmon fillets
- 2 tablespoons olive oil
- 2 tablespoons fresh lemon juice
- 2 cloves garlic, minced
- 1 tablespoon fresh dill, chopped
- Salt and pepper, to taste
- Lemon slices, for garnish

Instructions

- Preheat your oven to 375°F (190°C). Line a baking sheet with parchment paper or lightly grease it with olive oil.
- In a small bowl, mix together the olive oil, lemon juice, minced garlic, chopped dill, salt, and pepper.
- Place the salmon fillets on the prepared baking sheet. Brush each fillet with the lemon-dill mixture, coating them evenly.
- Place a lemon slice on top of each salmon fillet for added flavor.
- Bake the salmon in the preheated oven for 12-15 minutes, or until the salmon is cooked through and flakes easily with a fork.
- Once done, remove the salmon from the oven and garnish with fresh dill sprigs.
- Serve the baked salmon hot with your favorite side dishes.

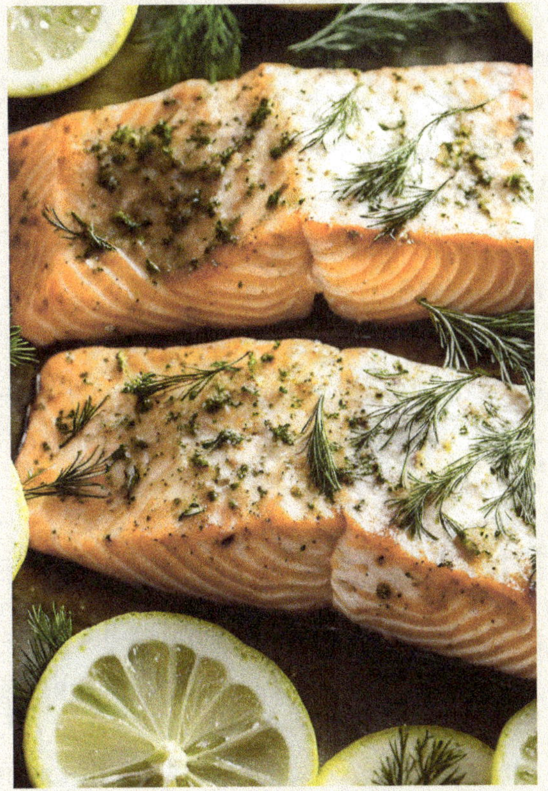

Preparation Time : 10 min

Total Time : 20 min

Servings : 4

Nutritional Info

- Calories: 280 kcal
- Protein: 25g
- Fat: 18g
- Carbohydrates: 2g
- Fiber: 0.5g

QUINOA AND VEGETABLE STUFFED PEPPERS

Ingredients

- 4 large bell peppers, any color
- 1 cup quinoa, rinsed
- 2 cups vegetable broth
- 1 tablespoon olive oil
- 1 onion, diced
- 2 cloves garlic, minced
- 1 zucchini, diced
- 1 carrot, diced
- 1 cup diced tomatoes
- 1 teaspoon dried oregano
- Salt and pepper to taste

Instructions

- Preheat oven to 375°F (190°C).
- Cook quinoa: In a saucepan, combine quinoa and vegetable broth. Bring to a boil, then simmer covered for 15 minutes until cooked.
- Prepare vegetables: Heat olive oil in a skillet. Add onion and garlic, cook until softened (about 5 mins). Then add zucchini and carrot, cook for another 5 mins until tender.
- Mix: Stir in diced tomatoes, oregano, cooked quinoa, salt, and pepper. Cook for 2-3 more minutes.
- Prepare peppers: Cut the tops off the bell peppers, remove seeds and membranes. Place in a baking dish.
- Fill peppers: Spoon quinoa and vegetable mixture into each pepper.
- Optional: Sprinkle shredded mozzarella cheese on top.
- Bake: Cover dish with foil, bake for 25-30 mins until peppers are tender.
- Serve hot and enjoy!

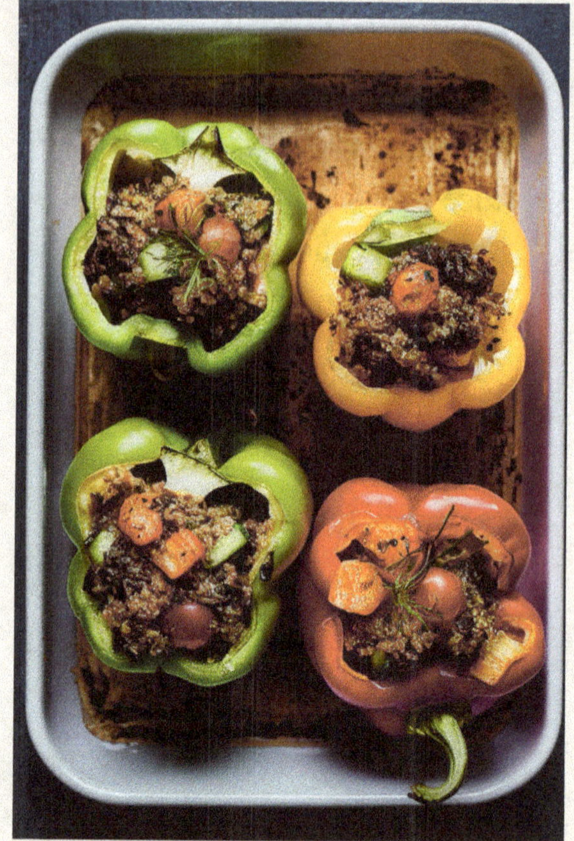

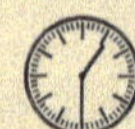 **Preparation Time : 20 min**

 **Total Time : 1 hour**

Servings : 4

Nutritional Info

- Calories: 295 kcal
- Total Fat: 7g
- Saturated Fat: 1g
- Cholesterol: 0mg
- Sodium: 460mg

TURMERIC CHICKEN AND RICE

Ingredients

- 1 lb boneless, skinless chicken breasts, cut into bite-sized pieces
- 2 cups white or brown rice
- 1 tablespoon olive oil
- 1 onion, chopped
- 3 cloves garlic, minced
- 1 tablespoon ground turmeric
- 1 teaspoon ground cumin
- 1 teaspoon ground coriander
- Salt and pepper to taste
- 3 cups chicken broth
- 1 cup frozen peas

Instructions

- Heat olive oil in a large skillet over medium heat. Add chopped onion and minced garlic, sauté until softened.
- Add chicken pieces to the skillet, cook until browned on all sides.
- Stir in ground turmeric, cumin, and coriander, coating the chicken evenly.
- Add rice to the skillet, stirring to combine with the chicken and spices.
- Pour chicken broth into the skillet, bring to a boil.
- Reduce heat to low, cover, and simmer for 20-25 minutes or until rice is cooked and liquid is absorbed.
- Stir in frozen peas, cover, and cook for an additional 5 minutes until peas are heated through.
- Garnish with chopped cilantro before serving.

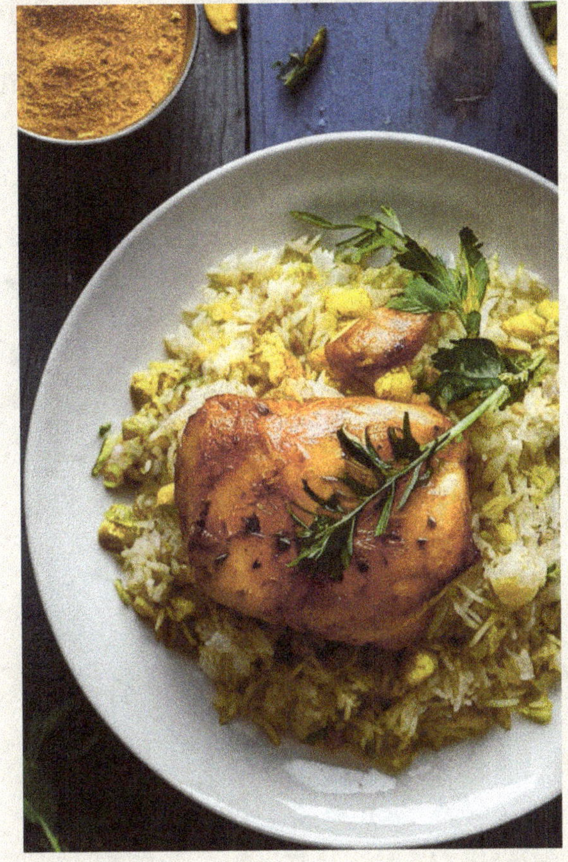

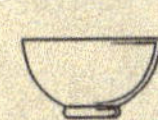
Preparation Time : 10 min

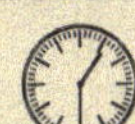
Total Time : 35 min

Servings : 4

Nutritional Info

- Calories: 400 kcal
- Protein: 30g
- Carbohydrates: 45g
- Fat: 10g
- Fiber: 4g

SWEET POTATO AND BLACK BEAN ENCHILADAS

Ingredients

- 2 medium sweet potatoes, peeled and diced
- 1 can (15 oz) black beans, drained and rinsed
- 1 cup corn kernels (fresh or frozen)
- 1 bell pepper, diced
- 1 small onion, diced
- 2 cloves garlic, minced
- 1 teaspoon ground cumin
- 1 teaspoon chili powder
- Salt and pepper, to taste
- 8 small corn tortillas
- 1 cup enchilada sauce
- 1 cup shredded cheese

Instructions

- Preheat oven to 375°F (190°C). Grease a baking dish.
- In a skillet over medium heat, cook sweet potatoes until soft, about 5-7 minutes.
- Add onion, bell pepper, and garlic. Cook until tender, about 5 minutes.
- Stir in black beans, corn, cumin, chili powder, salt, and pepper. Cook for 2-3 minutes.
- Warm tortillas in the microwave for 30 seconds.
- Spoon filling onto each tortilla. Roll up and place seam-side down in the baking dish.
- Pour enchilada sauce over the top. Sprinkle cheese evenly.
- Cover with foil and bake for 20 minutes.
- Remove foil and bake for 5-10 more minutes, until cheese melts.
- Garnish with cilantro if desired before serving.

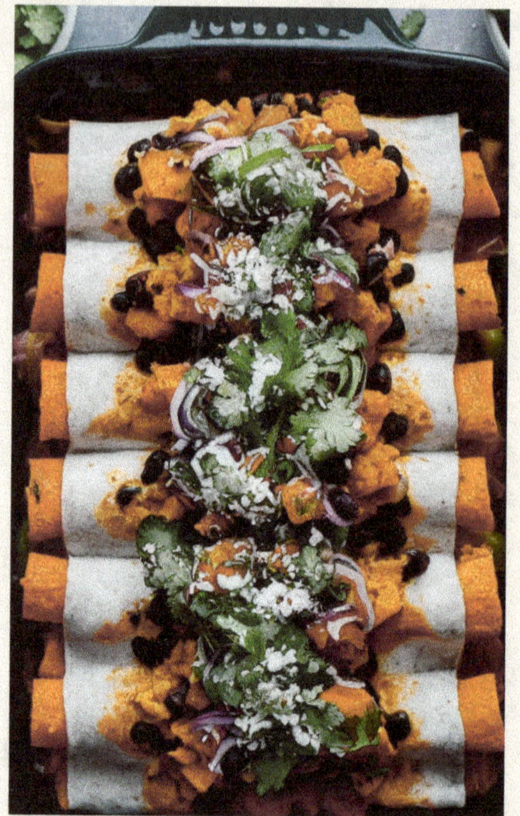

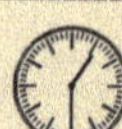 **Preparation Time : 15 min**

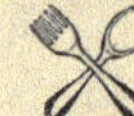 **Total Time : 35 min**

Servings : 4

Nutritional Info

- Calories: 380
- Total Fat: 10g
- Saturated Fat: 5g
- Cholesterol: 20mg
- Sodium: 680mg
- Total Carbohydrates: 59g

ZUCCHINI NOODLES WITH PESTO

Ingredients

- 4 medium zucchinis, spiralized
- 1 cup fresh basil leaves
- 1/4 cup pine nuts
- 2 cloves garlic
- 1/4 cup grated Parmesan cheese
- 1/4 cup olive oil
- Salt and pepper to taste

Instructions

- In a food processor, combine basil leaves, pine nuts, garlic, and Parmesan cheese. Pulse until finely chopped.
- With the processor running, slowly drizzle in the olive oil until the mixture forms a smooth paste. Season with salt and pepper to taste.
- In a large skillet over medium heat, add the spiralized zucchini noodles. Cook for 2-3 minutes until slightly softened but still crisp.
- Add the pesto sauce to the skillet with the zucchini noodles and toss until well coated.
- Serve immediately, garnished with sliced cherry tomatoes if desired.

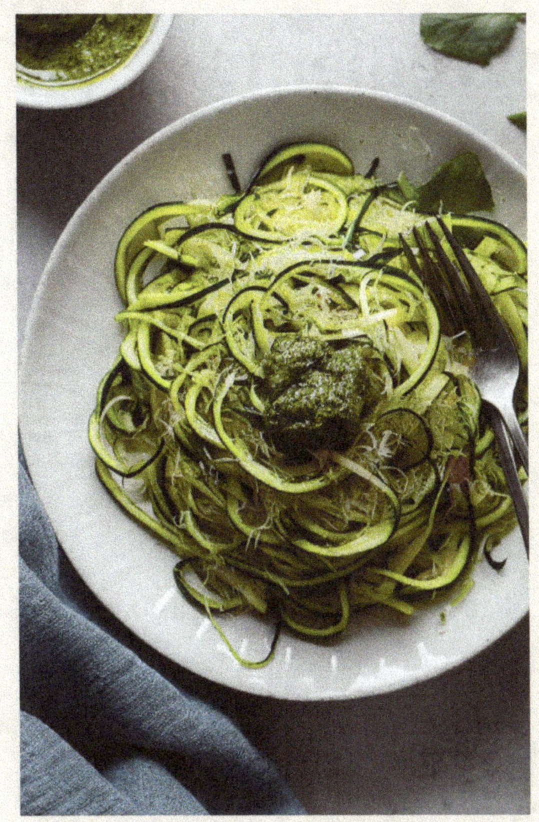

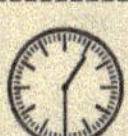 **Preparation Time : 10 min**

 **Total Time : 15 min**

Servings : 4

Nutritional Info

- Calories: 180 kcal
- Protein: 5g
- Fat: 16g
- Carbohydrates: 7g
- Fiber: 2g

HERB-ROASTED CHICKEN AND VEGETABLES

Ingredients

- 4 bone-in, skin-on chicken thighs
- 2 cups baby potatoes, halved
- 2 cups carrots, peeled and sliced into sticks
- 1 cup Brussels sprouts, halved
- 2 tablespoons olive oil
- 2 cloves garlic, minced
- 1 teaspoon dried thyme
- 1 teaspoon dried rosemary
- 1 teaspoon dried oregano
- Salt and pepper to taste

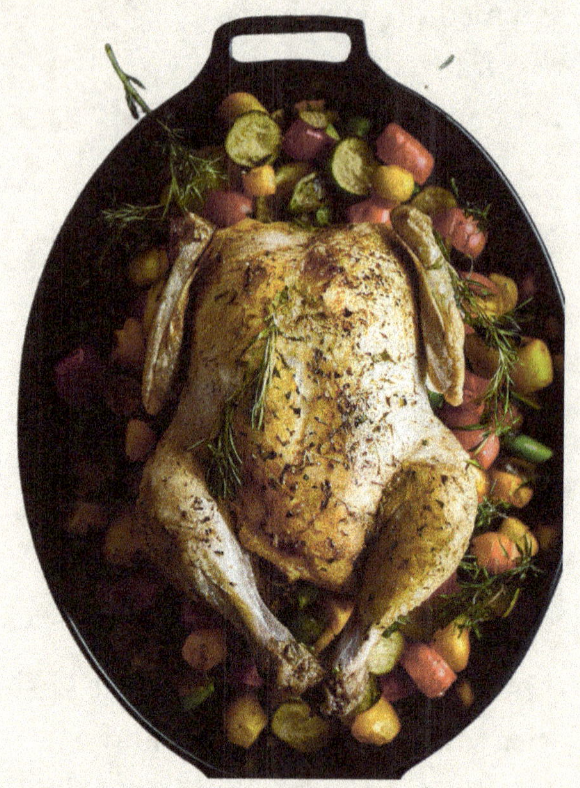

Instructions

- Preheat your oven to 400°F (200°C).
- In a large mixing bowl, combine the chicken thighs, potatoes, carrots, Brussels sprouts, olive oil, minced garlic, dried thyme, dried rosemary, dried oregano, salt, and pepper. Toss until everything is evenly coated.
- Transfer the chicken and vegetable mixture to a baking sheet lined with parchment paper or aluminum foil, arranging everything in a single layer.
- Roast in the preheated oven for 35-40 minutes or until the chicken is cooked through and the vegetables are tender and golden brown.
- Serve hot, garnished with fresh herbs if desired.

Preparation Time : 15 min

Total Time : 55 min

Servings : 4

Nutritional Info

- Calories: 380 kcal
- Total Fat: 20g
- Saturated Fat: 5g
- Trans Fat: 0g
- Cholesterol: 120mg
- Sodium: 210mg

GINGER-GARLIC SHRIMP STIR-FRY

Ingredients

- 1 lb shrimp, peeled and deveined
- 2 tablespoons olive oil
- 3 cloves garlic, minced
- 1 tablespoon fresh ginger, minced
- 1 red bell pepper, thinly sliced
- 1 yellow bell pepper, thinly sliced
- 1 cup snow peas
- 1/4 cup low-sodium soy sauce
- 2 tablespoons honey
- 2 green onions, chopped

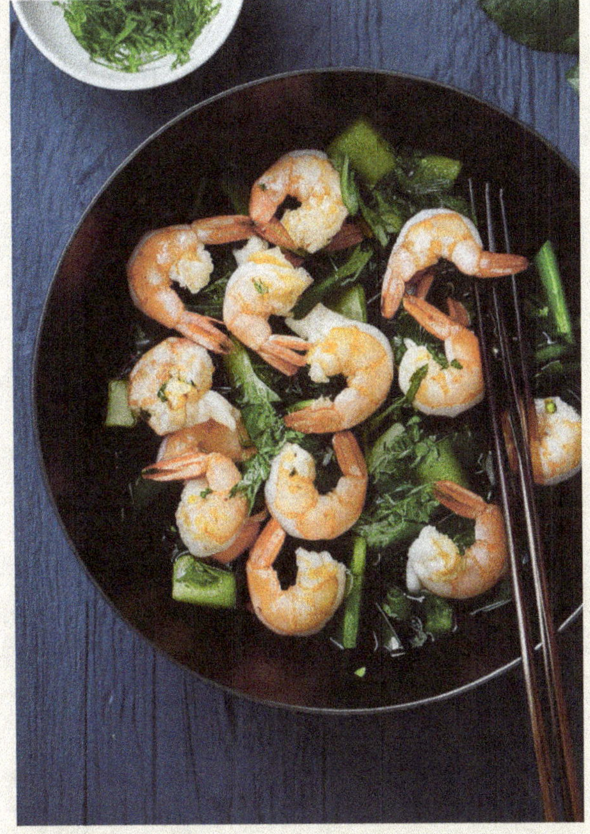

Instructions

- In a large pan, heat olive oil over medium-high heat.
- Add garlic and ginger, sauté for 1-2 minutes until fragrant.
- Add shrimp and cook for 3-4 minutes until pink and cooked through.
- Stir in bell peppers and snow peas, cook for an additional 2-3 minutes.
- In a small bowl, mix soy sauce and honey. Pour over the shrimp and vegetables, stirring to combine.
- Cook for another 1-2 minutes, until the sauce has thickened slightly.
- Remove from heat and sprinkle with chopped green onions.
- Serve over cooked rice.

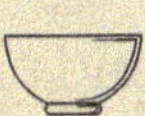 **Preparation Time : 15 min**

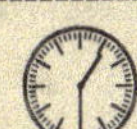 **Total Time : 25 min**

 **Servings : 4**

Nutritional Info

- Calories: 280
- Protein: 25g
- Fat: 10g
- Carbohydrates: 20g
- Fiber: 3g

LENTIL AND SPINACH CURRY

Ingredients

- 1 cup dried lentils
- 2 cups fresh spinach, chopped
- 1 onion, finely chopped
- 2 cloves garlic, minced
- 1 tablespoon curry powder
- 1 teaspoon ground cumin
- 1 teaspoon ground coriander
- 1 can (14 ounces) diced tomatoes
- 1 can (14 ounces) coconut milk
- Salt and pepper, to taste

Instructions

- Rinse the lentils under cold water until the water runs clear. Drain well.
- In a large pot or skillet, heat some oil over medium heat. Add the chopped onion and minced garlic, and sauté until softened and fragrant, about 3-4 minutes.
- Stir in the curry powder, ground cumin, and ground coriander. Cook for another minute until the spices are toasted and fragrant.
- Add the rinsed lentils, diced tomatoes (with their juices), and coconut milk to the pot. Stir to combine.
- Bring the mixture to a boil, then reduce the heat to low. Cover and simmer for about 20-25 minutes, or until the lentils are tender and cooked through.
- Stir in the chopped spinach and cook for an additional 2-3 minutes, until the spinach is wilted.
- Season with salt and pepper to taste.
- Serve the lentil and spinach curry hot over cooked rice. Garnish with fresh cilantro.

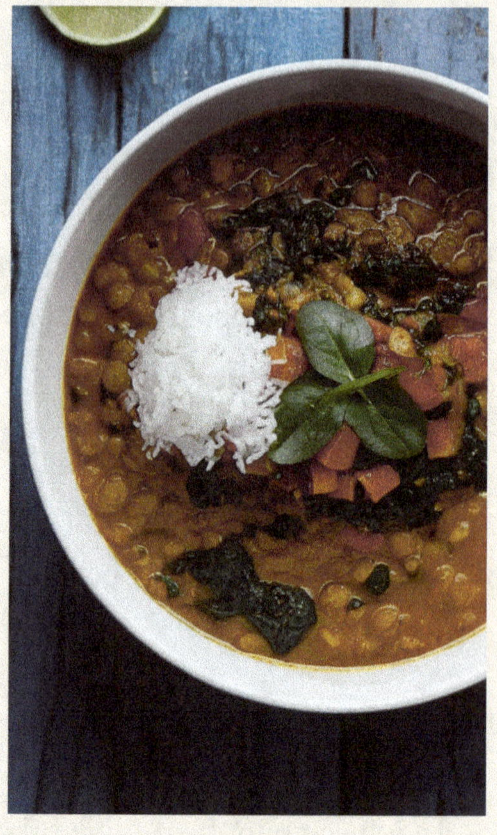

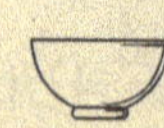 **Preparation Time : 10 min**

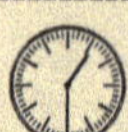 **Total Time : 35 min**

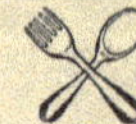 **Servings : 4**

Nutritional Info

- Calories: 320 kcal
- Protein: 15g
- Carbohydrates: 40g
- Fat: 12g
- Fiber: 14g

ROASTED CAULIFLOWER STEAKS

Ingredients

- 1 large head of cauliflower
- 2-3 tablespoons olive oil
- Salt and pepper to taste
- Optional: your favorite seasoning blend (such as garlic powder, smoked paprika, or cumin)

Instructions

- Preheat your oven to 425°F (220°C).
- Remove the outer leaves of the cauliflower and trim the stem end to create a flat base.
- Place the cauliflower head on a cutting board and slice it vertically into 1-inch thick slices, creating "steaks." You should get 2-3 steaks from one head of cauliflower.
- Place the cauliflower steaks on a baking sheet lined with parchment paper or aluminum foil.
- Drizzle olive oil over the cauliflower steaks and use your hands to rub it evenly on both sides.
- Season the cauliflower steaks with salt, pepper, and any optional seasoning blend of your choice.
- Roast in the preheated oven for 25-30 minutes, flipping halfway through, until the cauliflower is tender and golden brown on the edges.

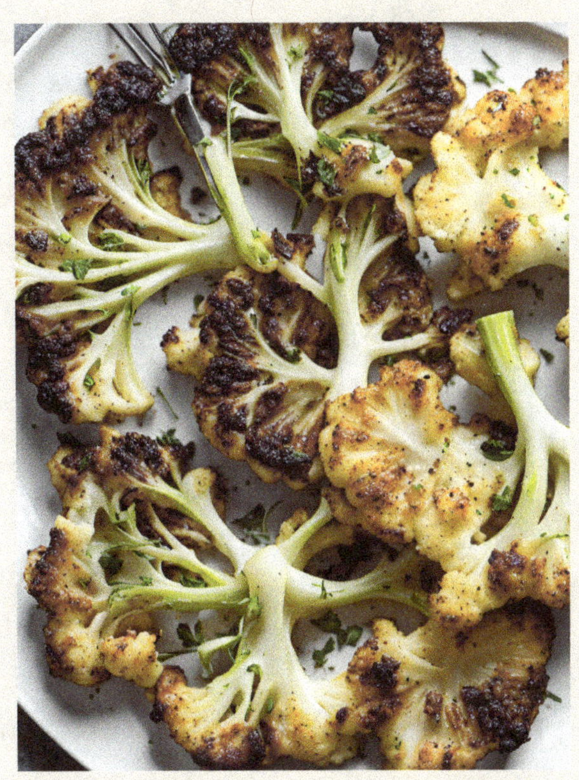

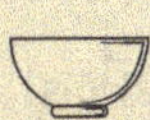 **Preparation Time : 10 min**

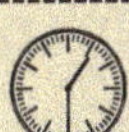 **Total Time : 35 min**

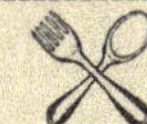 **Servings : 2-3**

Nutritional Info

- Calories: 120 kcal
- Protein: 5g
- Fat: 9g
- Carbohydrates: 10g
- Fiber: 5g

BAKED COD WITH TOMATO AND OLIVE RELISH

Ingredients

- 4 cod fillets (about 6 oz each)
- 1 cup cherry tomatoes, halved
- 1/4 cup Kalamata olives, chopped
- 2 tablespoons olive oil
- 2 cloves garlic, minced
- 1 tablespoon fresh lemon juice
- Salt and pepper to taste
- Fresh parsley, chopped (for garnish)

Instructions

- Preheat the oven to 400°F (200°C).
- Place the cod fillets on a baking dish lined with parchment paper.
- In a small bowl, mix the cherry tomatoes, olives, olive oil, garlic, lemon juice, salt, and pepper.
- Spoon the tomato and olive mixture over the cod fillets.
- Bake for 15-20 minutes, or until the fish is cooked through and flakes easily with a fork.
- Garnish with fresh parsley before serving.

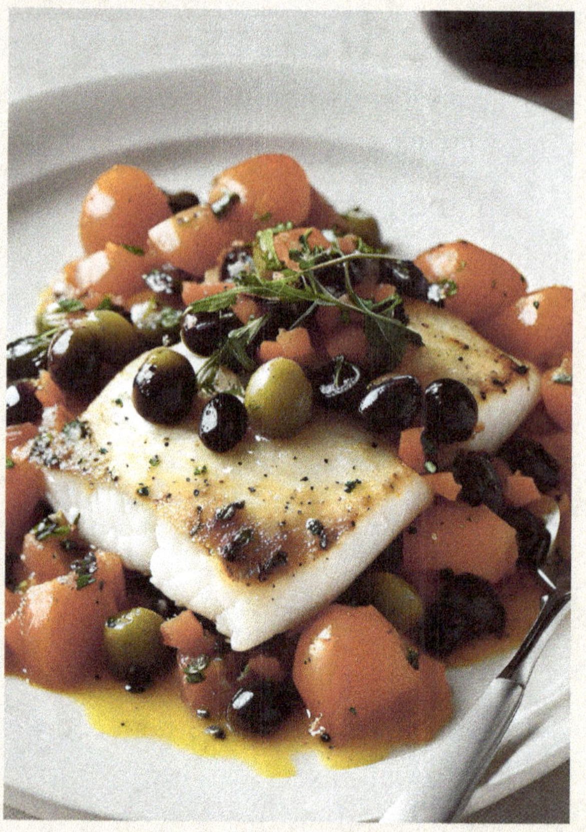

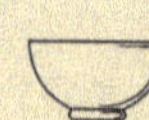 **Preparation Time : 10 min**

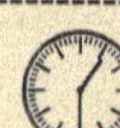 **Total Time : 25 min**

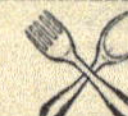 **Servings : 4**

Nutritional Info

- Calories: 300
- Protein: 30g
- Fat: 14g
- Carbohydrates: 8g
- Fiber: 2g

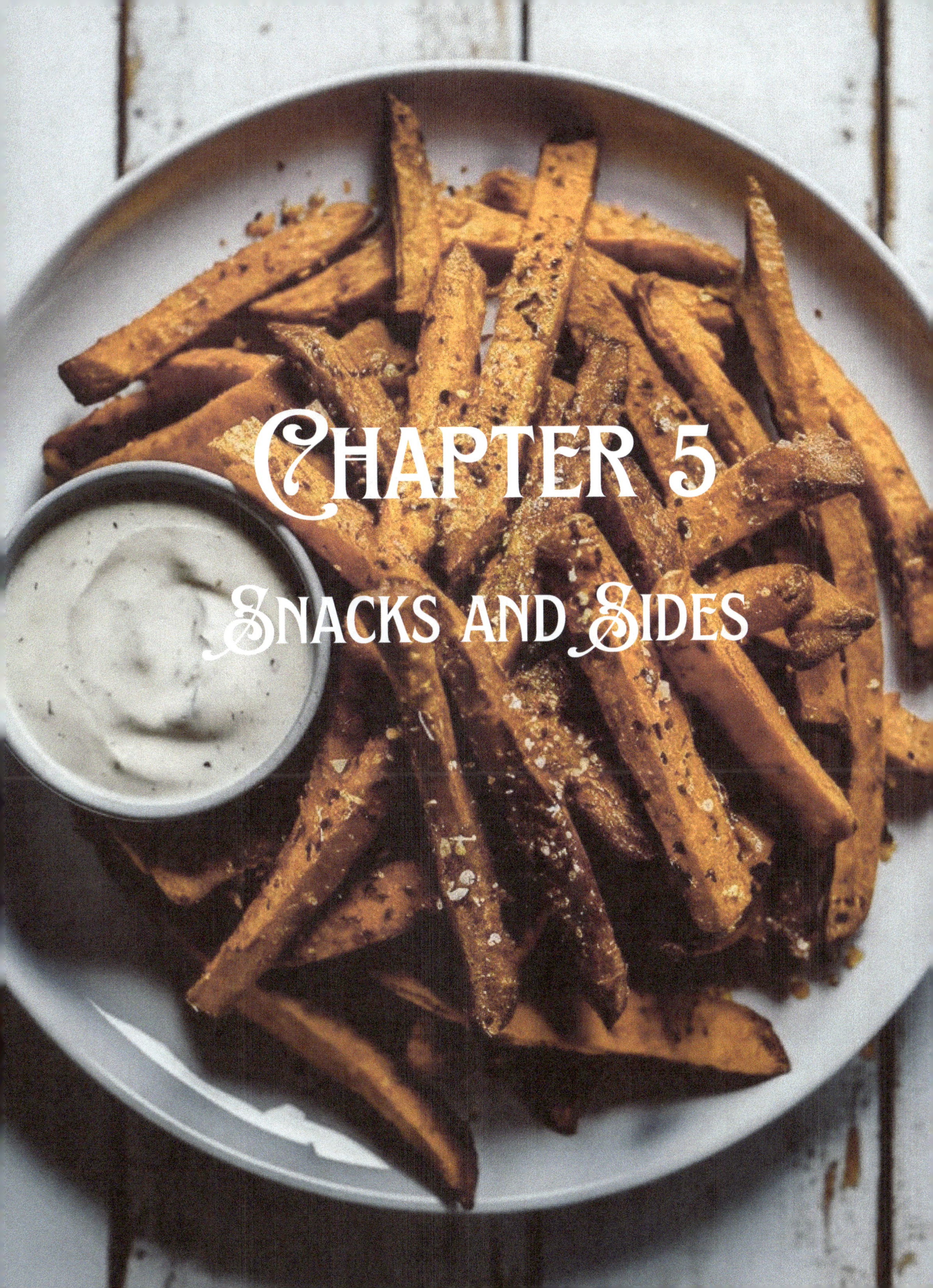
Chapter 5
Snacks and Sides

EDAMAME WITH SEA SALT

Ingredients

- 2 cups frozen edamame in pods
- 1 tablespoon sea salt (or to taste)
- Water for boiling

Instructions

- Fill a large pot with water and bring it to a boil over high heat.
- Once the water is boiling, add the frozen edamame pods to the pot.
- Boil for 5 minutes, or until the edamame pods are tender and easily open when squeezed.
- Drain the edamame in a colander and rinse under cold water to stop the cooking process.
- Transfer the edamame to a bowl and sprinkle with sea salt. Toss to evenly coat the pods with the salt.
- Serve immediately as a snack or appetizer.
- To eat, simply squeeze the edamame beans out of the pods and discard the pods.

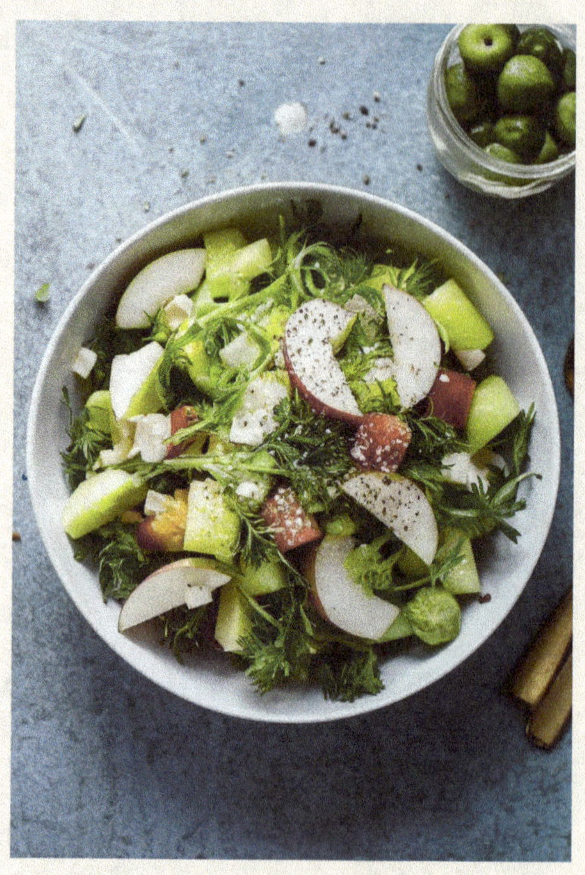

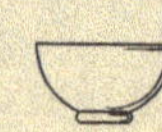 **Preparation Time : 5 min**

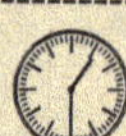 **Total Time : 15 min**

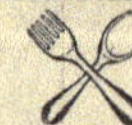 **Servings : 4**

Nutritional Info

- Calories: 120
- Protein: 12g
- Carbohydrates: 10g
- Fat: 5g
- Fiber: 4g
- Sodium: 150mg

SPICED SWEET POTATO FRIES

Ingredients

- 2 large sweet potatoes
- 1 teaspoon paprika
- 1/2 teaspoon garlic powder
- 1/2 teaspoon onion powder
- 1/2 teaspoon ground cumin
- 1/4 teaspoon cayenne pepper (optional)
- Salt and pepper to taste

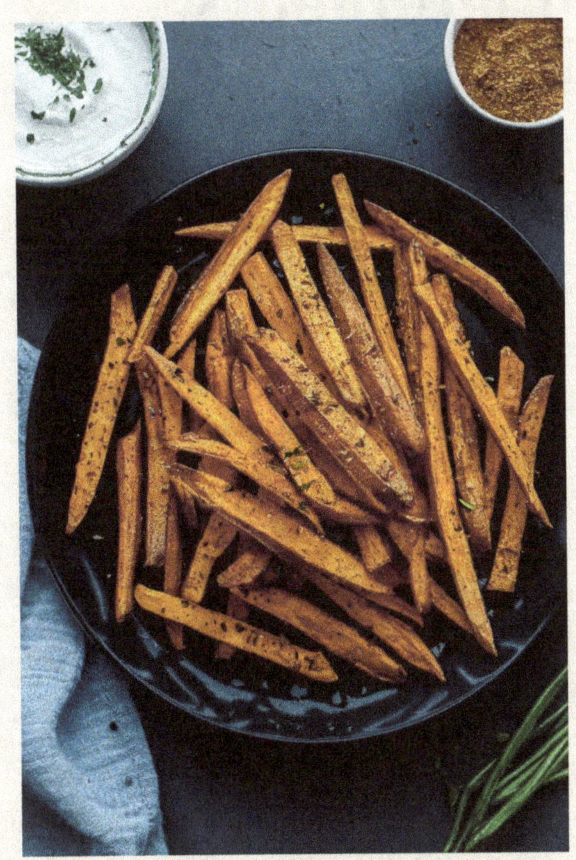

Instructions

- Preheat Oven: Preheat oven to 425°F (220°C). Line a baking sheet with parchment paper or spray with cooking spray.
- Cut Sweet Potatoes: Peel and cut sweet potatoes into thin fries.
- Season: Mix paprika, garlic powder, onion powder, cumin, cayenne pepper (if using), salt, and pepper in a large bowl. Add sweet potatoes and toss to coat.
- Bake: Spread fries on the baking sheet in a single layer. Bake for 20-25 minutes, turning halfway through, until golden and crispy.
- Serve: Let cool slightly and enjoy!

Preparation Time : 10 min

Total Time : 35 min

Servings : 4

Nutritional Info

- Calories: 120
- Protein: 2g
- Carbohydrates: 27g
- Fiber: 4g
- Fat: 0.5g

GUACAMOLE WITH VEGGIE STICKS

Ingredients

- 2 ripe avocados
- 1 small tomato, diced
- 1/4 cup red onion, finely chopped
- 1 jalapeño pepper, seeded and minced (optional for spice)
- 2 tablespoons fresh cilantro, chopped
- 1 tablespoon lime juice
- Salt and pepper to taste

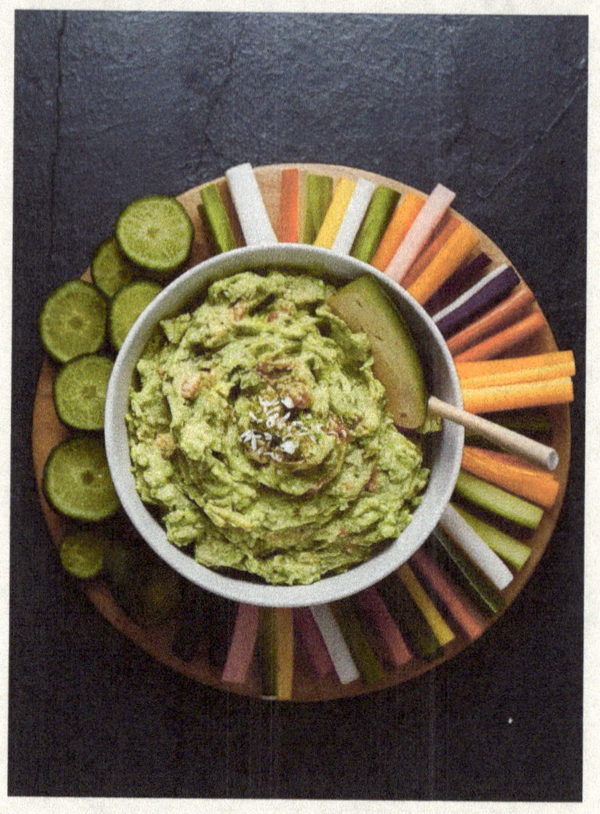

Instructions

- Cut the avocados in half, remove the pits, and scoop the flesh into a mixing bowl.
- Mash the avocados with a fork until smooth or until your desired consistency is reached.
- Add the diced tomato, chopped red onion, minced jalapeño pepper (if using), chopped cilantro, and lime juice to the bowl with the mashed avocado.
- Season with salt and pepper to taste.
- Stir all the ingredients until well combined.
- Taste and adjust seasoning if necessary.
- Transfer the guacamole to a serving bowl and garnish with additional cilantro if desired.
- Serve the guacamole with assorted vegetable sticks for dipping.

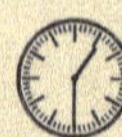 **Preparation Time : 10 min**

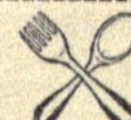 **Total Time : 10 min**

Servings : 4

Nutritional Info

- Calories: 120
- Total Fat: 10g
- Saturated Fat: 1.5g
- Sodium: 250mg
- Total Carbohydrates: 8g
- Dietary Fiber: 6g

ROASTED CHICKPEAS

Ingredients

- 1 can (15 oz) chickpeas, drained and rinsed
- 1 tablespoon olive oil
- 1 teaspoon paprika
- 1 teaspoon garlic powder
- 1/2 teaspoon salt
- 1/4 teaspoon black pepper

Instructions

- Preheat Oven: Preheat your oven to 400°F (200°C).
- Dry Chickpeas: Pat the chickpeas dry with paper towels.
- Season Chickpeas: In a bowl, mix chickpeas with olive oil, paprika, garlic powder, salt, and pepper.
- Bake: Spread chickpeas on a baking sheet. Bake for 35-40 minutes, shaking the pan halfway through.
- Cool: Let cool for a few minutes before serving.

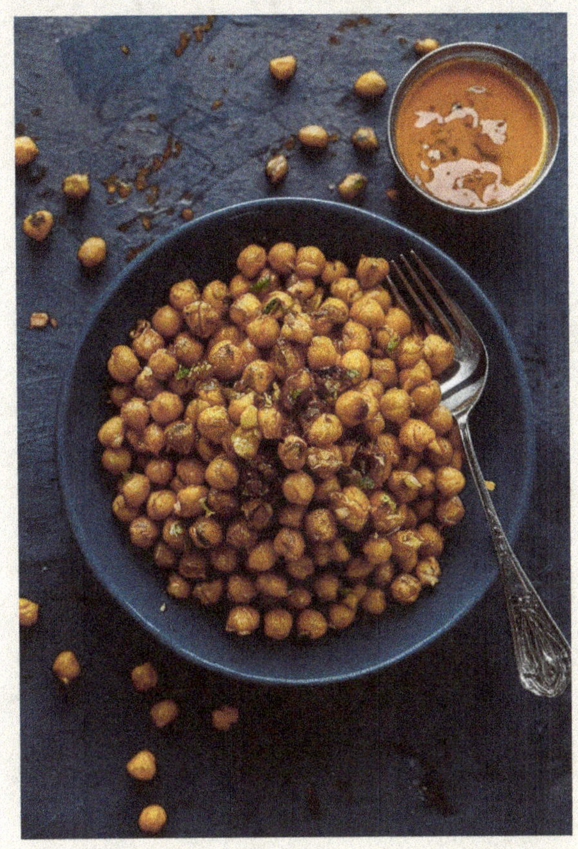

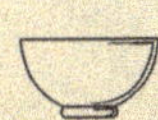 Preparation Time : 10 min

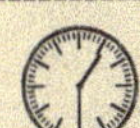 Total Time : 50 min

 Servings : 4

Nutritional Info

- Calories: 120
- Protein: 6g
- Fat: 2g
- Carbohydrates: 20g
- Fiber: 6g

BAKED KALE CHIPS

Ingredients

- 1 bunch of kale
- 1 tablespoon olive oil (optional)
- 1 teaspoon sea salt

Instructions

- Preheat oven to 300°F (150°C).
- Prepare kale: Wash and dry kale. Tear into bite-sized pieces, removing stems.
- Season: Toss kale with olive oil (if using) and salt.
- Bake: Spread kale on a baking sheet in a single layer. Bake for 20 minutes, until edges are brown.
- Cool and serve: Let cool for a few minutes to crisp up. Enjoy!

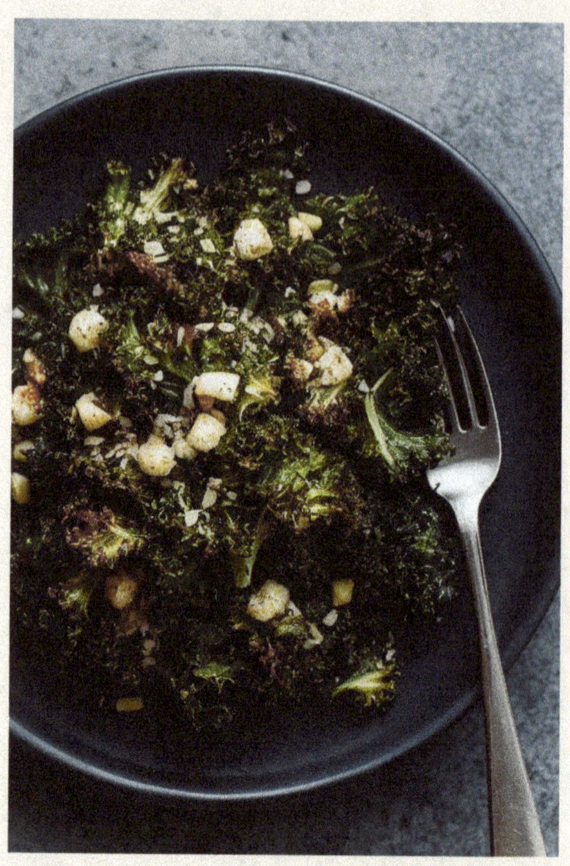

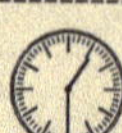 **Preparation Time : 10 min**

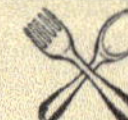 **Total Time : 30 min**

Servings : 4

Nutritional Info

- Calories: 50
- Total Fat: 2g (with olive oil)
- Saturated Fat: 0g
- Cholesterol: 0mg
- Sodium: 200mg
- Total Carbohydrates: 8g

SPICED NUTS

Ingredients

- 2 cups mixed nuts (such as almonds, walnuts, and cashews)
- 1 tablespoon olive oil
- 1 tablespoon honey or maple syrup
- 1 teaspoon ground cinnamon
- 1/2 teaspoon ground nutmeg
- 1/4 teaspoon ground cloves
- 1/4 teaspoon salt

Instructions

- Preheat your oven to 350°F (175°C) and line a baking sheet with parchment paper.
- In a large bowl, combine the mixed nuts, olive oil, honey or maple syrup, cinnamon, nutmeg, cloves, and salt. Toss until the nuts are evenly coated.
- Spread the coated nuts in a single layer on the prepared baking sheet.
- Bake for 10-15 minutes, stirring occasionally, until the nuts are toasted and fragrant.
- Remove from the oven and let cool completely before serving or storing in an airtight container.

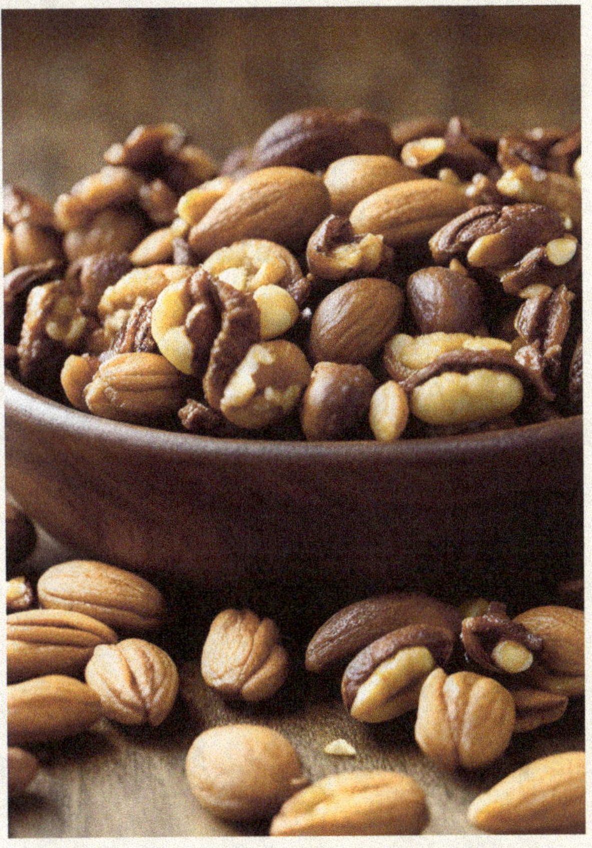

Preparation Time : 5 min

Total Time : 20 min

Servings : 1/4 cup

Nutritional Info

- Calories: 180
- Protein: 5g
- Fat: 15g
- Carbohydrates: 8g
- Fiber: 2g

CRUNCHY CELERY AND APPLE SALAD

Ingredients

- 4 stalks of celery, thinly sliced
- 2 large apples (Granny Smith or Honeycrisp), cored and diced
- 1/4 cup walnuts, chopped (optional)
- 1/4 cup raisins (optional)
- 2 tablespoons lemon juice
- 1/2 teaspoon salt
- 1/4 teaspoon black pepper
- 1 tablespoon olive oil (optional)

Instructions

- Wash and thinly slice the celery stalks.
- Core and dice the apples into bite-sized pieces.
- In a large mixing bowl, combine the sliced celery and diced apples.
- If using, add the chopped walnuts and raisins to the bowl.
- Drizzle the lemon juice over the salad mixture to prevent the apples from browning.
- Season with salt and black pepper.
- Add the olive oil, if desired, for a richer flavor.
- Toss all ingredients together until well combined.
- Garnish with chopped parsley if desired.
- Serve the salad immediately to maintain its crunchiness.

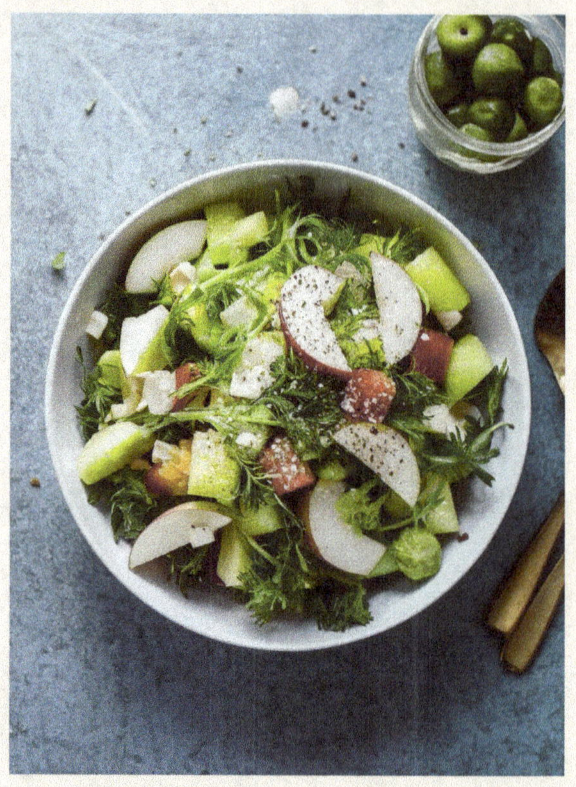

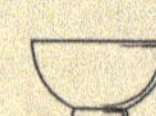
Preparation Time : 15 min

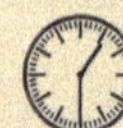
Total Time : 15 min

Servings : 4

Nutritional Info

- Calories: 80
- Protein: 1g
- Carbohydrates: 18g
- Fat: 1g
- Fiber: 4g

MIXED BERRY SALAD

Ingredients

- 2 cups mixed berries (such as strawberries, blueberries, raspberries)
- 2 tablespoons honey
- 1 tablespoon balsamic vinegar
- 1/4 cup fresh mint leaves, chopped
- 1/4 cup crumbled feta cheese (optional)
- Salt and pepper to taste

Instructions

- Wash the berries and pat them dry. Slice the strawberries if they are large.
- In a small bowl, whisk together the honey and balsamic vinegar.
- In a large bowl, combine the mixed berries and chopped mint leaves.
- Drizzle the honey-balsamic dressing over the berries and gently toss to coat.
- Season with salt and pepper to taste.
- Sprinkle the crumbled feta cheese on top, if using.
- Serve immediately.

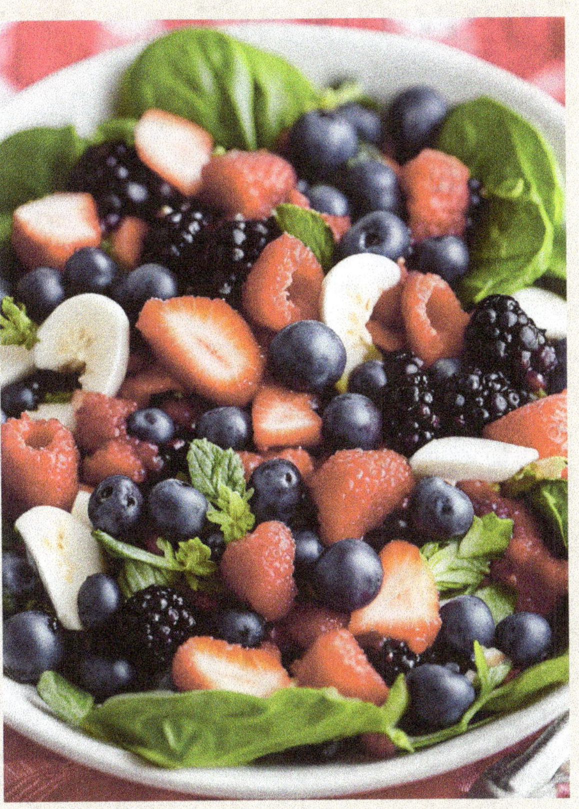

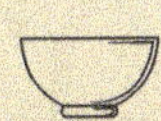 **Preparation Time : 10 min**

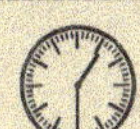 **Total Time : 10 min**

 **Servings : 4**

Nutritional Info

- Calories: 90
- Total Fat: 1g
- Cholesterol: 0mg
- Sodium: 20mg
- Total Carbohydrates: 22g

ALMOND BUTTER AND APPLE SLICES

Ingredients

- 2 medium-sized apples
- 1/4 cup almond butter
- Optional: drizzle of honey or sprinkle of cinnamon

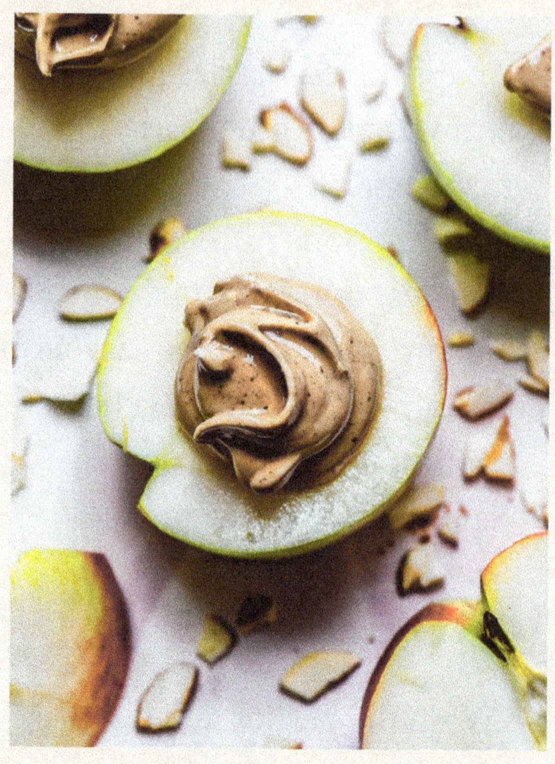

Instructions

- Wash and core the apples. Slice them into thin rounds or wedges.
- Spread almond butter on one side of each apple slice.
- Optional: Drizzle honey or sprinkle cinnamon over the almond butter.
- Serve immediately and enjoy!

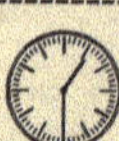 **Preparation Time : 5 min**

 **Total Time : 5 min**

Servings : 4

Nutritional Info

- Calories: Approximately 180 kcal
- Total Fat: 11g
- Saturated Fat: 1g
- Trans Fat: 0g
- Cholesterol: 0mg
- Sodium: 5mg

MARINATED MUSHROOM SKEWERS

Ingredients

- 1 lb (450g) button mushrooms, cleaned and stems trimmed
- 2 tbsp olive oil
- 3 tbsp balsamic vinegar
- 2 cloves garlic, minced
- 1 tsp dried thyme
- 1 tsp dried rosemary
- Salt and pepper to taste

Instructions

- Mix olive oil, balsamic vinegar, garlic, thyme, rosemary, salt, and pepper in a bowl.
- Add mushrooms and toss to coat. Let sit for 10 minutes.
- If using wooden skewers, soak them in water for 10 minutes.
- Thread mushrooms onto skewers.
- Preheat grill to medium-high.
- Grill skewers for 5-7 minutes per side, until mushrooms are tender.
- Remove from grill and enjoy warm.

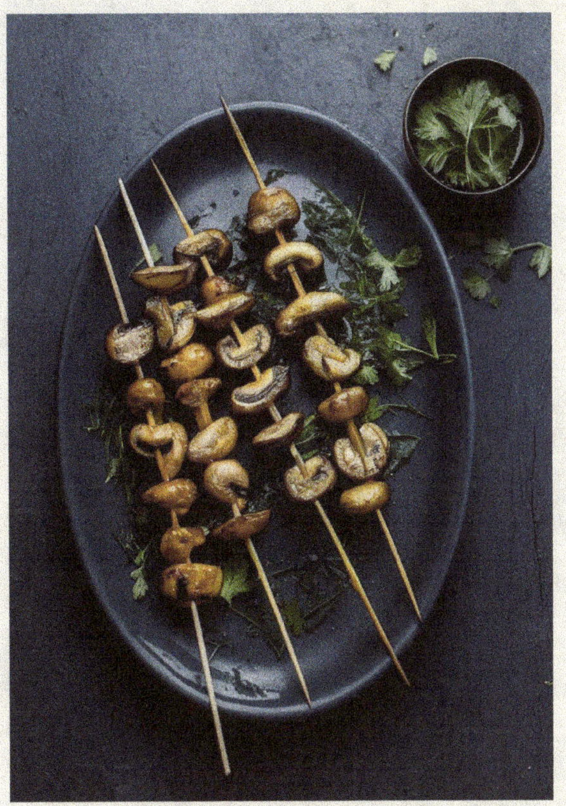

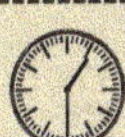 **Preparation Time : 10 min**

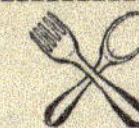 **Total Time : 20 min**

Servings : 4

Nutritional Info

- Calories: 80
- Protein: 2g
- Carbohydrates: 6g
- Fat: 5g
- Fiber: 2g
- Sugar: 3g

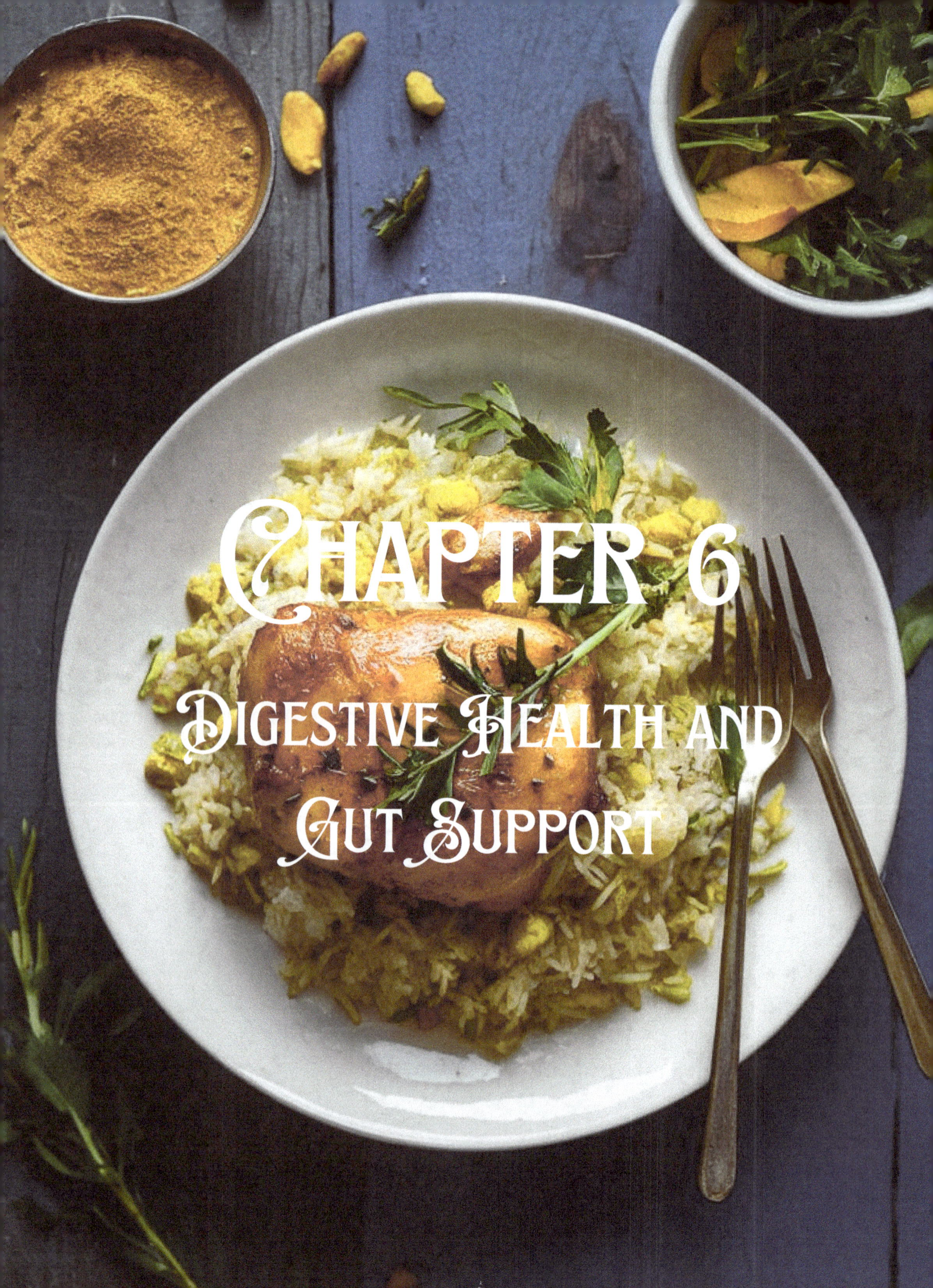

Chapter 6
Digestive Health and Gut Support

BEEF AND BROCCOLI STIR-FRY

Ingredients

- 1 lb (450g) lean beef steak, thinly sliced
- 2 cups broccoli florets
- 1 red bell pepper, thinly sliced
- 1 onion, thinly sliced
- 3 cloves garlic, minced
- 2 tbsp low-sodium soy sauce
- 1 tbsp oyster sauce
- 1 tbsp sesame oil
- 1 tbsp cornstarch
- 1 tsp fresh ginger, grated
- 2 tbsp vegetable oil
- Salt and pepper, to taste

Instructions

- In a bowl, mix soy sauce, oyster sauce, sesame oil, cornstarch, and grated ginger.
- Add beef to the marinade and let it sit for 10 minutes.
- Heat vegetable oil in a skillet or wok over medium-high heat.
- Add minced garlic and cook until fragrant, about 30 seconds.
- Add marinated beef and cook until browned, about 3 minutes. Remove beef.
- In the same skillet, add more oil if needed, then add broccoli, bell pepper, and onion. Cook for 3-4 minutes until tender-crisp.
- Return beef to the skillet, stir together, and cook for 2 minutes to heat through.
- Season with salt and pepper.
- Garnish with sesame seeds and green onions if desired.
- Serve hot over rice or noodles.

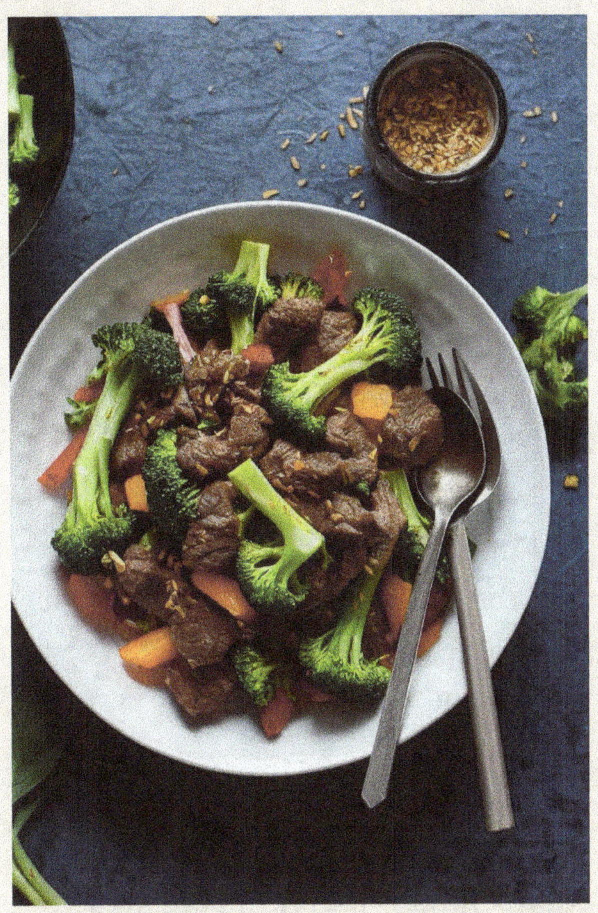

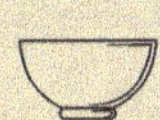 **Preparation Time : 15 min**

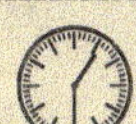 **Total Time : 30 min**

 **Servings : 4**

Nutritional Info

- Calories: 250
- Protein: 25g
- Carbohydrates: 12g
- Fat: 11g
- Fiber: 4g

TURKEY MEATBALLS WITH ZOODLES

Ingredients

- 1 lb ground turkey
- 1/4 cup grated Parmesan cheese
- 1 large egg
- 2 cloves garlic, minced
- 1/4 cup chopped parsley
- 1 tsp dried oregano
- 1/2 tsp salt
- 1/4 tsp black pepper
- 4 medium zucchinis, spiralized
- 2 tbsp olive oil
- 1 clove garlic, minced
- Salt and pepper to taste

Instructions

- Mix turkey, Parmesan, egg, minced garlic, parsley, oregano, salt, and pepper in a bowl.
- Shape into 1-inch meatballs.
- Heat a large skillet over medium-high heat with a bit of olive oil.
- Cook meatballs until browned and cooked through, about 10-12 minutes.
- Remove meatballs from the skillet.
- In the same skillet, heat 2 tbsp olive oil over medium heat.
- Add minced garlic and cook for 1 minute.
- Add spiralized zucchini and cook for 3-5 minutes until tender.
- Season with salt and pepper.
- Return meatballs to the skillet and add marinara sauce.
- Heat until warm.
- Serve meatballs and sauce over zoodles.

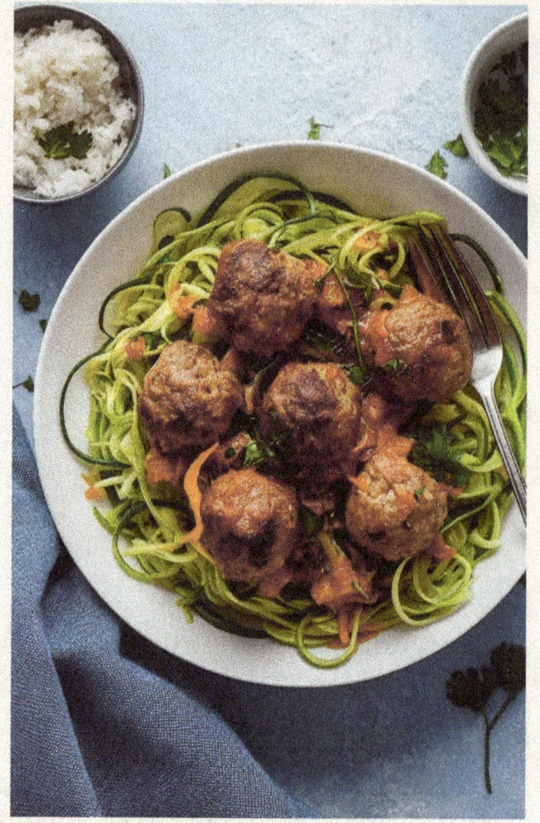

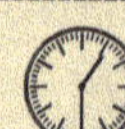 **Preparation Time : 20 min**

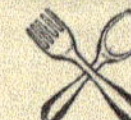 **Total Time : 45 min**

Servings : 4

Nutritional Info

- Calories: 250
- Protein: 30g
- Carbohydrates: 10g
- Fat: 10g
- Fiber: 3g

VEGGIE STIR-FRY WITH TOFU

Ingredients

- 1 block (14 oz) firm tofu, cubed
- 2 tablespoons soy sauce (low sodium)
- 1 tablespoon olive oil
- 2 bell peppers, sliced
- 1 cup broccoli florets
- 1 cup snap peas
- 2 cloves garlic, minced
- 1 tablespoon fresh ginger, grated
- 2 tablespoons vegetable broth (low sodium)
- Salt and pepper to taste

Instructions

- Drain, pat dry, and cube the tofu. Toss with 1 tablespoon soy sauce.
- Heat olive oil in a large pan over medium-high heat. Cook tofu until golden brown, about 5-7 minutes. Remove from pan.
- In the same pan, add garlic and ginger, sauté for 30 seconds.
- Add bell peppers, broccoli, and snap peas. Stir-fry for 4-5 minutes until tender-crisp.
- Return tofu to pan. Add 1 tablespoon soy sauce and vegetable broth. Stir and cook for 2-3 minutes.
- Season with salt and pepper. Serve warm.

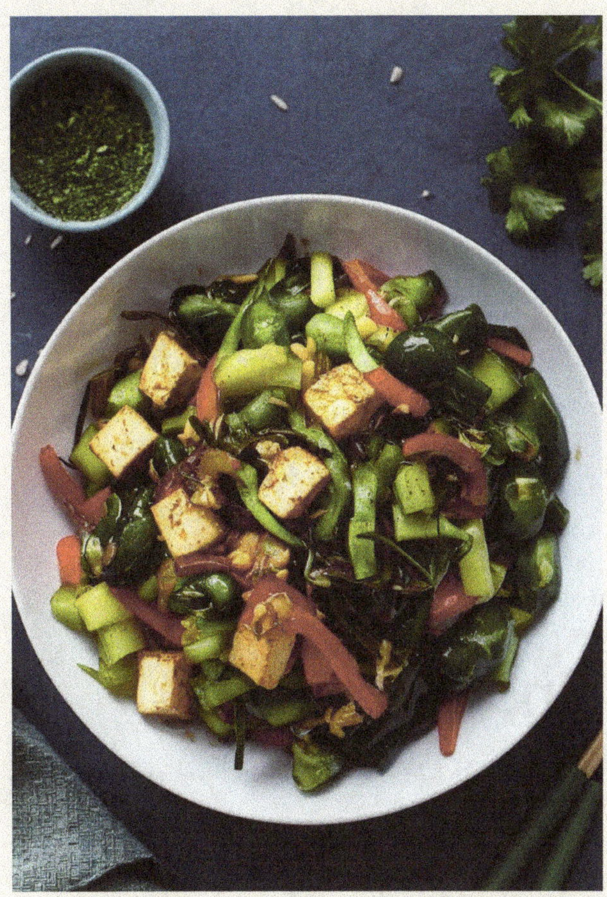

Preparation Time : 10 min

Total Time : 20 min

Servings : 4

Nutritional Info

- Calories: 180
- Protein: 12g
- Carbohydrates: 16g
- Fat: 8g
- Fiber: 5g

HERB-CRUSTED CHICKEN BREAST

Ingredients

- 4 boneless, skinless chicken breasts
- 2 tablespoons olive oil
- 1/4 cup fresh parsley, chopped
- 1/4 cup fresh basil, chopped
- 1/4 cup fresh thyme, chopped
- 2 cloves garlic, minced
- 1 teaspoon salt
- 1/2 teaspoon black pepper
- 1 teaspoon lemon zest

Instructions

- Preheat Oven: Preheat your oven to 400°F (200°C).
- Prepare Herb Mixture: In a small bowl, combine the chopped parsley, basil, thyme, minced garlic, salt, black pepper, and lemon zest.
- Prepare Chicken: Pat the chicken breasts dry with paper towels. Rub each breast with olive oil, ensuring they are evenly coated.
- Coat with Herbs: Press the herb mixture onto both sides of each chicken breast, making sure they are well coated.
- Bake Chicken: Place the chicken breasts on a baking sheet lined with parchment paper or in a lightly greased baking dish.
- Cook: Bake in the preheated oven for 25 minutes, or until the internal temperature of the chicken reaches 165°F (74°C) and the exterior is golden brown.
- Rest and Serve: Let the chicken rest for 5 minutes before serving to allow the juices to redistribute.

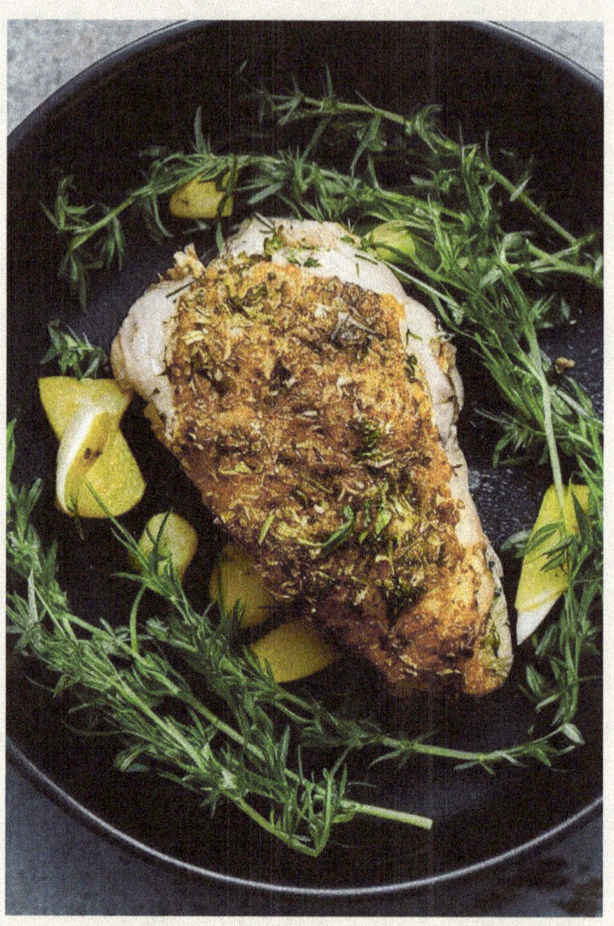

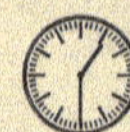 **Preparation Time : 15 min**

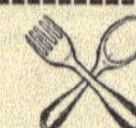 **Total Time : 40 min**

Servings : 4

Nutritional Info

- Calories: 220
- Protein: 28g
- Carbohydrates: 2g
- Fat: 11g

SPAGHETTI SQUASH WITH MARINARA SAUCE

Ingredients

- 1 medium spaghetti squash
- 2 cups marinara sauce
- 2 tablespoons olive oil
- Salt and pepper to taste

Instructions

- Preheat oven to 400°F (200°C).
- Cut spaghetti squash in half lengthwise and remove seeds.
- Drizzle olive oil over cut sides of squash and season with salt and pepper.
- Place squash halves cut-side down on a baking sheet.
- Roast squash in oven for 35-40 minutes, until tender.
- While squash is roasting, heat marinara sauce in a saucepan on medium heat.
- Once squash is done, remove from oven and let cool slightly.
- Use a fork to scrape flesh into spaghetti-like strands onto a plate.
- Pour heated marinara sauce over spaghetti squash.
- Serve hot and enjoy!

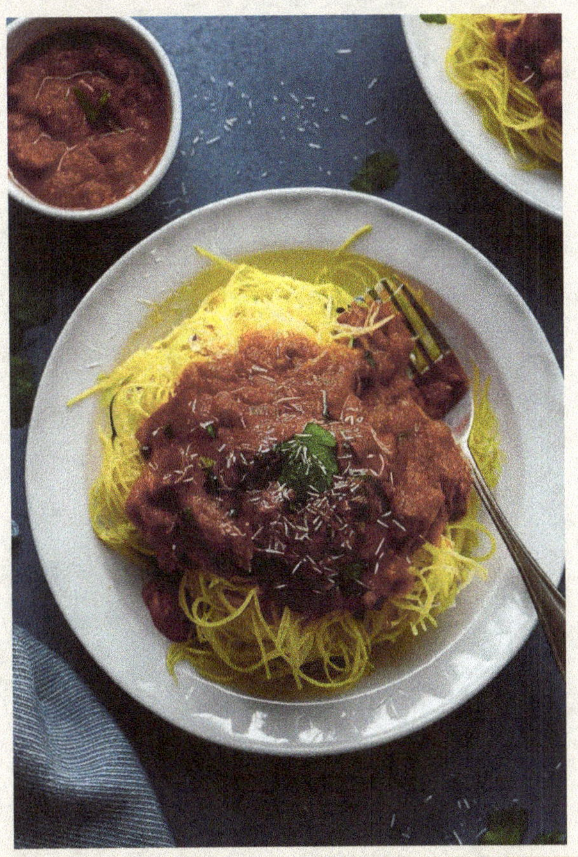

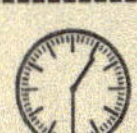 **Preparation Time : 10 min**

 **Total Time : 50 min**

Servings : 4

Nutritional Info

- Calories: 150
- Total Fat: 6g
- Total Carbohydrates: 24g
- Protein: 3g

BALSAMIC GLAZED CHICKEN BREAST

Ingredients

- 4 boneless, skinless chicken breasts
- 1/2 cup balsamic vinegar
- 2 tablespoons honey
- 2 cloves garlic, minced
- 1 teaspoon dried thyme
- Salt and pepper
- 1 tablespoon olive oil

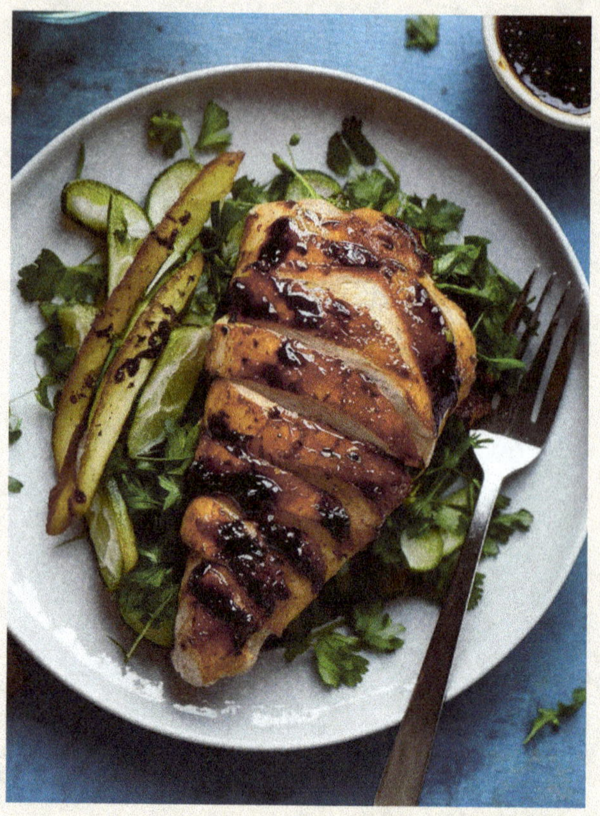

Instructions

- Mix balsamic vinegar, honey, minced garlic, and dried thyme in a bowl.
- Pour over chicken breasts and let sit for 10 minutes.
- Heat olive oil in a skillet over medium-high heat.
- Remove chicken from marinade (save marinade) and season with salt and pepper.
- Cook chicken for 5 minutes on each side until browned.
- Pour the reserved marinade into the skillet.
- Cook for another 10 minutes, turning chicken to coat with glaze, until chicken is cooked through (165°F internal temperature).
- Let chicken rest for 5 minutes.
- Drizzle with remaining glaze from the skillet.

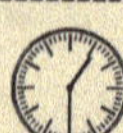 **Preparation Time : 10 min**

 **Total Time : 30 min**

Servings : 4

Nutritional Info

- Calories: 200
- Protein: 30g
- Fat: 4g
- Carbohydrates: 8g

GRILLED VEGETABLE KEBABS

Ingredients

- 1 red bell pepper, cut into chunks
- 1 yellow bell pepper, cut into chunks
- 1 zucchini, sliced into rounds
- 1 red onion, cut into chunks
- 8 cherry tomatoes
- 8 button mushrooms
- 2 tablespoons olive oil
- 1 teaspoon dried oregano
- 1 teaspoon dried basil
- Salt and pepper to taste

Instructions

- Wash and cut the vegetables as indicated.
- If using wooden skewers, soak them in water for at least 10 minutes to prevent burning.
- In a large bowl, combine the olive oil, dried oregano, dried basil, salt, and pepper.
- Add the cut vegetables to the bowl and toss to coat them evenly with the marinade.
- Thread the marinated vegetables onto the skewers, alternating between different types of vegetables for a colorful presentation.
- Preheat your grill to medium-high heat.
- Place the kebabs on the preheated grill.
- Grill for about 10-15 minutes, turning occasionally, until the vegetables are tender and slightly charred.
- Remove the kebabs from the grill and serve immediately.

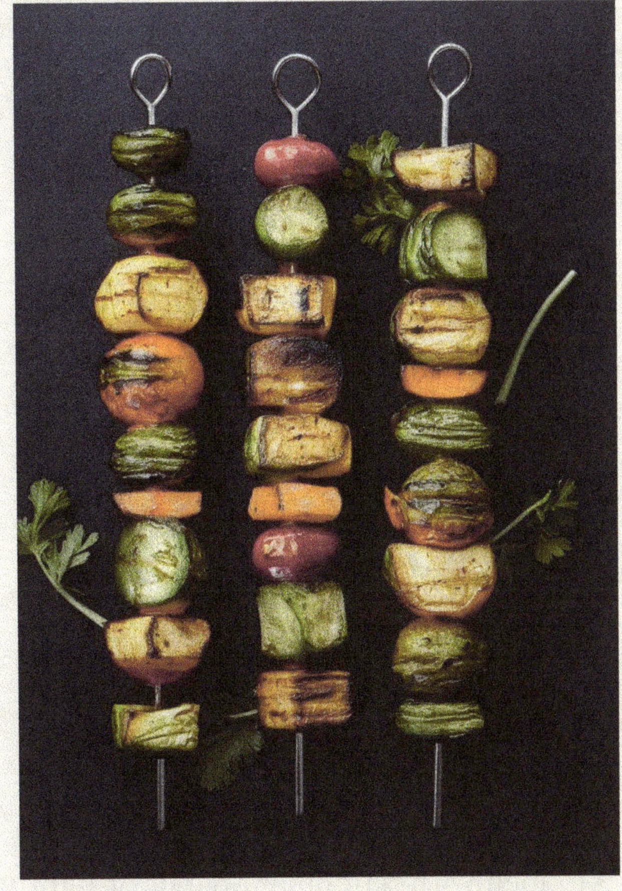

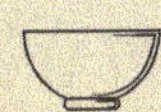 **Preparation Time : 20 min**

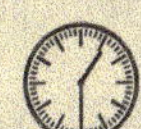 **Total Time : 35min**

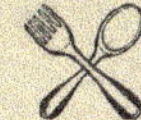 **Servings : 4**

Nutritional Info

- Calories: 90
- Protein: 3g
- Carbohydrates: 15g
- Fat: 3g
- Fiber: 5g

BAKED COD WITH LEMON AND DILL

Ingredients

- 4 cod fillets (about 6 ounces each)
- 2 tablespoons olive oil
- 2 cloves garlic, minced
- 1 tablespoon fresh dill, chopped
- 1 lemon, thinly sliced
- Salt and pepper to taste

Instructions

- Preheat your oven to 375°F (190°C).
- Place the cod fillets on a baking dish lined with parchment paper or lightly greased.
- In a small bowl, mix together the olive oil, minced garlic, and chopped dill.
- Drizzle the olive oil mixture over the cod fillets, making sure they are evenly coated.
- Season the cod fillets with salt and pepper to taste.
- Place lemon slices on top of each cod fillet.
- Bake in the preheated oven for about 15-20 minutes, or until the cod is cooked through and flakes easily with a fork.
- Remove from the oven and serve hot, garnished with additional fresh dill if desired.

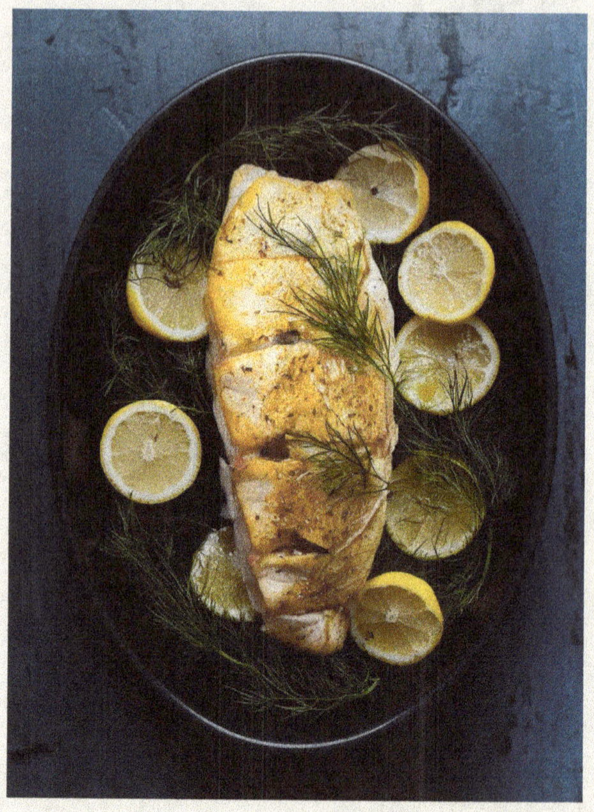

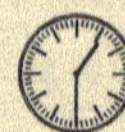 **Preparation Time : 10 min**

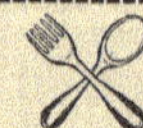 **Total Time : 30 min**

Servings : 4

Nutritional Info

- Calories: 150 kcal
- Protein: 25g
- Carbohydrates: 2g
- Fat: 4g
- Fiber: 0.5g
- Sugar: 0g

BAKED LEMON HERB SALMON

Ingredients

- 4 salmon fillets (about 6 oz each)
- 2 tablespoons olive oil
- 2 lemons (one for juice, one for slices)
- 3 cloves garlic, minced
- 2 tablespoons fresh parsley, chopped
- 1 tablespoon fresh dill, chopped
- 1 teaspoon salt
- 1/2 teaspoon black pepper

Instructions

- Preheat your oven to 400°F (200°C).
- Place the salmon fillets on a baking sheet lined with parchment paper.
- In a small bowl, mix the olive oil, juice of one lemon, minced garlic, chopped parsley, chopped dill, salt, and black pepper.
- Brush the marinade generously over each salmon fillet. Let it sit for about 10 minutes to allow the flavors to infuse.
- Slice the second lemon into thin rounds and place a couple of slices on top of each salmon fillet.
- Bake in the preheated oven for 20 minutes, or until the salmon is cooked through and flakes easily with a fork.
- Remove from the oven and transfer to plates. Serve immediately, optionally garnished with extra fresh herbs and lemon wedges.

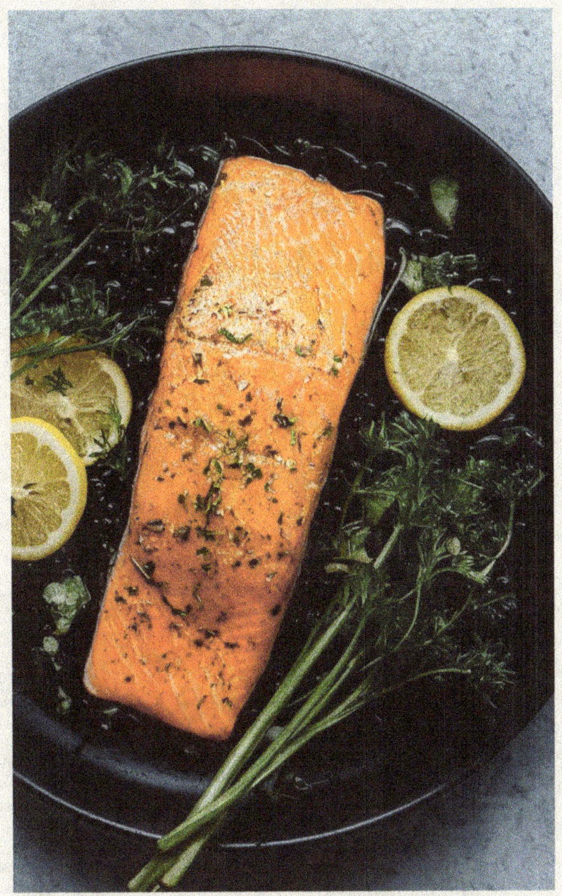

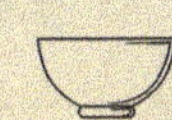 **Preparation Time : 10 min**

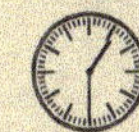 **Total Time : 30 min**

 **Servings : 4**

Nutritional Info

- Calories: 230
- Protein: 25g
- Fat: 14g
- Carbohydrates: 2g
- Fiber: 1g

Ingredients

- 1 lb large shrimp, peeled and deveined
- 2 cloves garlic, minced
- 2 tbsp olive oil
- 1 tbsp lemon juice
- 1 tsp smoked paprika
- Salt and pepper to taste
- Fresh parsley, chopped (for garnish)

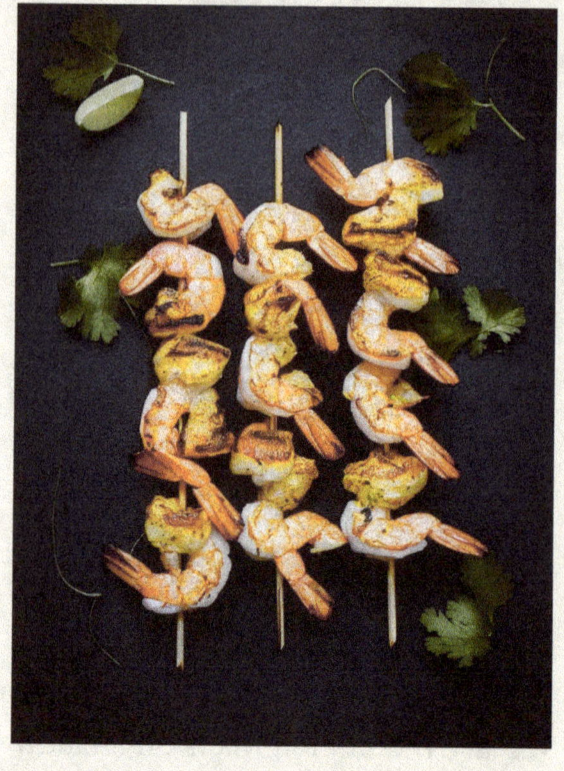

Instructions

- Marinate the Shrimp: In a large bowl, combine minced garlic, olive oil, lemon juice, smoked paprika, salt, and pepper. Add the shrimp and toss to coat. Let it marinate for 10 minutes.
- Prepare the Skewers: If using wooden skewers, soak them in water for 10 minutes to prevent burning. Thread the shrimp onto the skewers, leaving a little space between each shrimp.
- Preheat the Grill: Preheat the grill to medium-high heat.
- Grill the Shrimp: Place the shrimp skewers on the grill. Cook for 2-3 minutes per side, until the shrimp are opaque and cooked through.
- Serve: Remove the skewers from the grill and transfer to a serving platter. Garnish with chopped fresh parsley and lemon wedges. Serve immediately.

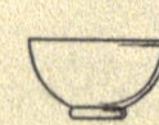 **Preparation Time : 15 min**

 **Total Time : 25 min**

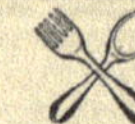 **Servings : 4**

Nutritional Info

- Calories: 150
- Protein: 23g
- Carbohydrates: 2g
- Fat: 6g
- Fiber: 0g

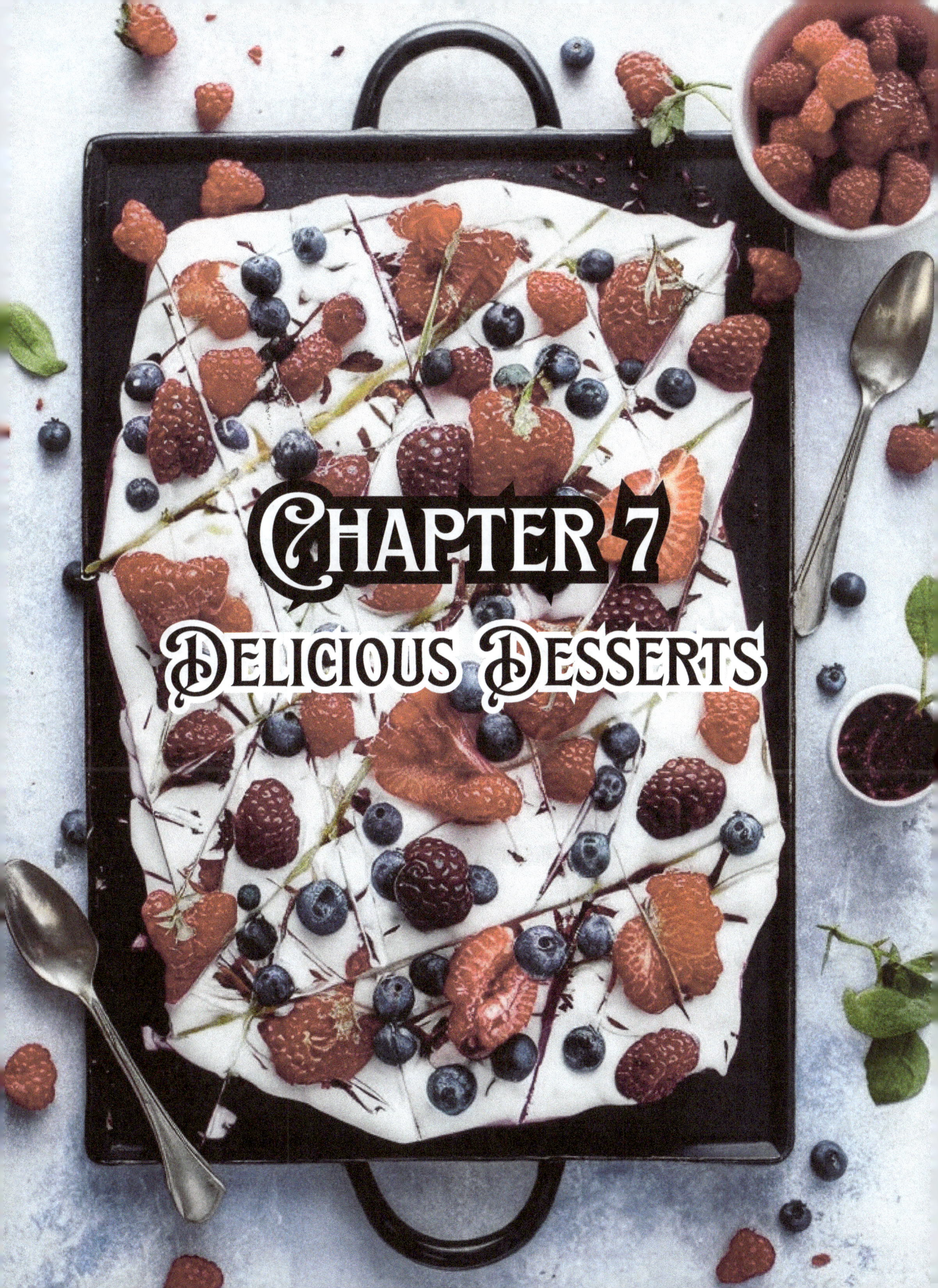

Chapter 7
Delicious Desserts

MIXED BERRY SORBET

Ingredients

- 3 cups mixed berries (such as strawberries, blueberries, raspberries)
- 1/4 cup honey or maple syrup (optional)
- 2 tablespoons lemon juice

Instructions

- Blend: Put the mixed berries, honey or maple syrup (if using), and lemon juice in a blender or food processor.
- Blend Again: Blend until smooth.
- Freeze: Pour the mixture into a shallow dish or pan. Cover and freeze for 3-4 hours, or until partially frozen.
- Scrape and Blend: Once partially frozen, scrape the mixture with a fork to break it up into icy flakes. Blend again until smooth.
- Freeze Again: Return the mixture to the dish or pan. Cover and freeze for another 2-3 hours, or until firm.
- Serve: Scoop the sorbet into bowls or glasses.
- Enjoy: Garnish with fresh mint leaves if desired, then serve and enjoy!

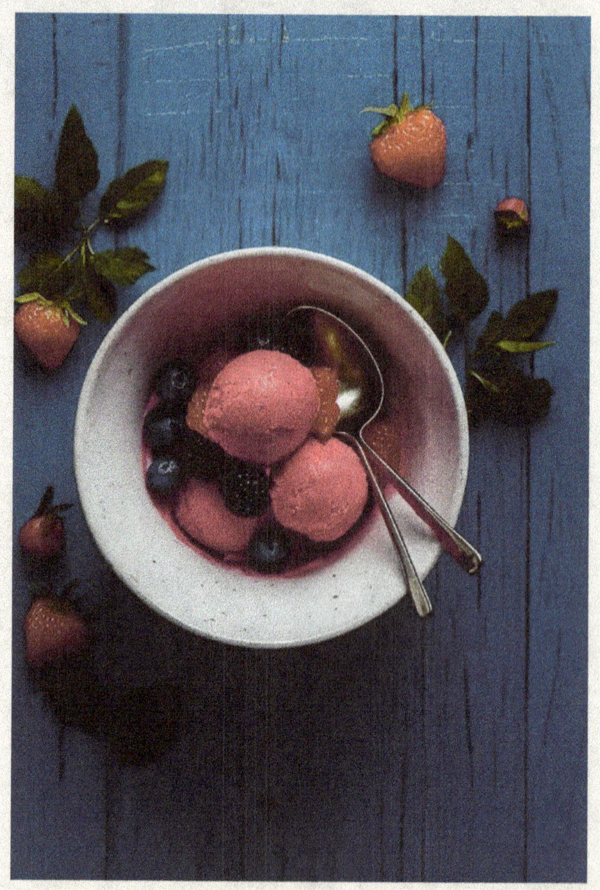

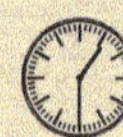 **Preparation Time : 10 min**

 **Total Time : 0 min**

Servings : 4

Nutritional Info

- Calories: Approximately 80 kcal
- Carbohydrates: Approximately 20 g
- Fiber: Approximately 3 g
- Sugars: Approximately 15 g
- Fat: Approximately 0 g

APPLE CINNAMON COMPOTE

Ingredients

- 4 medium apples, peeled, cored, and chopped
- 1 tablespoon lemon juice
- 1/4 cup water
- 2 tablespoons honey or maple syrup (optional)
- 1 teaspoon ground cinnamon
- 1/2 teaspoon vanilla extract (optional)

Instructions

- In a medium saucepan, combine the chopped apples, lemon juice, and water.
- Bring the mixture to a simmer over medium heat.
- Stir in the honey or maple syrup (if using), ground cinnamon, and vanilla extract (if using).
- Reduce the heat to low and let the mixture cook uncovered for about 15-20 minutes, or until the apples are soft and the liquid has thickened slightly, stirring occasionally.
- Once the apples are cooked to your desired consistency, remove the saucepan from the heat.
- Allow the compote to cool slightly before serving. You can serve it warm or chilled, depending on your preference.
- Enjoy the apple cinnamon compote on its own, or use it as a topping for yogurt, oatmeal, pancakes, or ice cream.

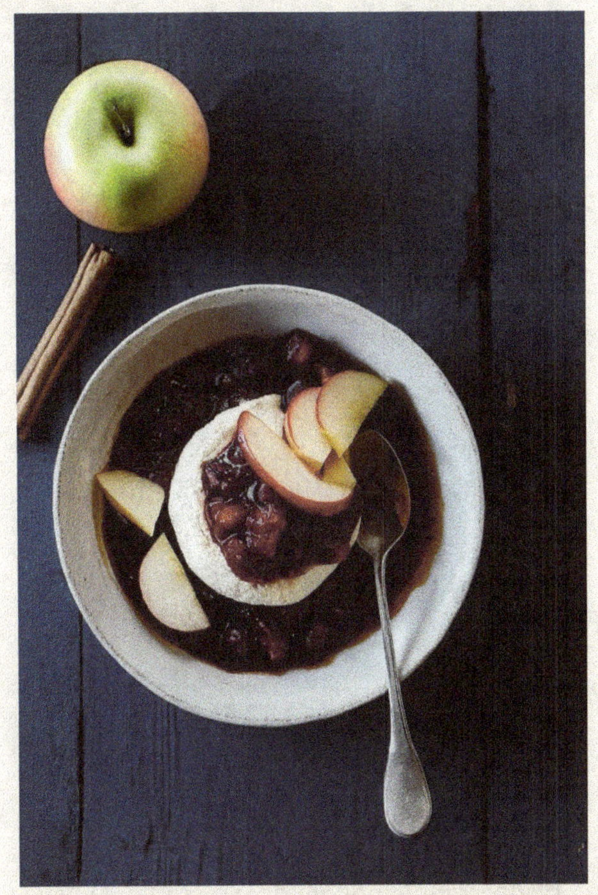

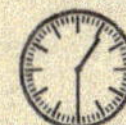 **Preparation Time : 10 min**

 **Total Time : 30 min**

Servings : 4

Nutritional Info

- Calories: 80 kcal
- Carbohydrates: 20 g
- Fiber: 4 g
- Sugars: 15 g
- Fat: 0 g
- Protein: 0 g

PEACH AND RASPBERRY CRUMBLE

Ingredients

- 1 ripe peach, sliced
- 1/2 cup fresh raspberries
- 1 tablespoon lemon juice
- 2 tablespoons granulated sugar (or sweetener of choice)
- 1/4 cup rolled oats
- 2 tablespoons all-purpose flour
- 1 tablespoon brown sugar
- 1/4 teaspoon ground cinnamon
- 2 tablespoons unsalted butter, chilled and cubed

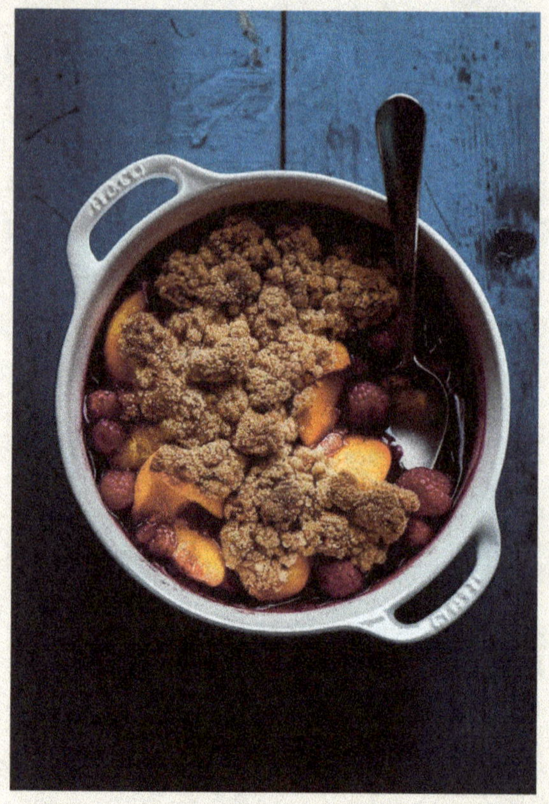

Instructions

- Preheat your oven to 375°F (190°C). Lightly grease a small baking dish or individual ramekins.
- In a bowl, toss together the sliced peach, raspberries, lemon juice, and granulated sugar until well combined. Transfer the fruit mixture to the prepared baking dish or ramekins, spreading it out evenly.
- In another bowl, mix together the rolled oats, all-purpose flour, brown sugar, and ground cinnamon.
- Using your fingers, incorporate the chilled cubed butter into the oat mixture until it resembles coarse crumbs.
- Sprinkle the oat mixture evenly over the fruit in the baking dish or ramekins.
- Place the baking dish or ramekins in the preheated oven and bake for about 25-30 minutes, or until the fruit is bubbly and the crumble topping is golden brown.
- Remove from the oven and let it cool for a few minutes before serving.
- Serve warm as is or with a scoop of vanilla frozen yogurt or a dollop of whipped cream, if desired.

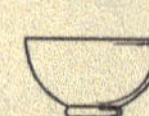 **Preparation Time : 15 min**

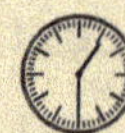 **Total Time : 45 min**

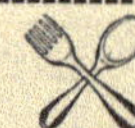 **Servings : 1**

Nutritional Info

- Calories: 250 kcal
- Carbohydrates: 40g
- Protein: 3g
- Fat: 10g
- Fiber: 5g

BAKED APPLES WITH CINNAMON

Ingredients

- 4 medium-sized apples
- 1 teaspoon ground cinnamon

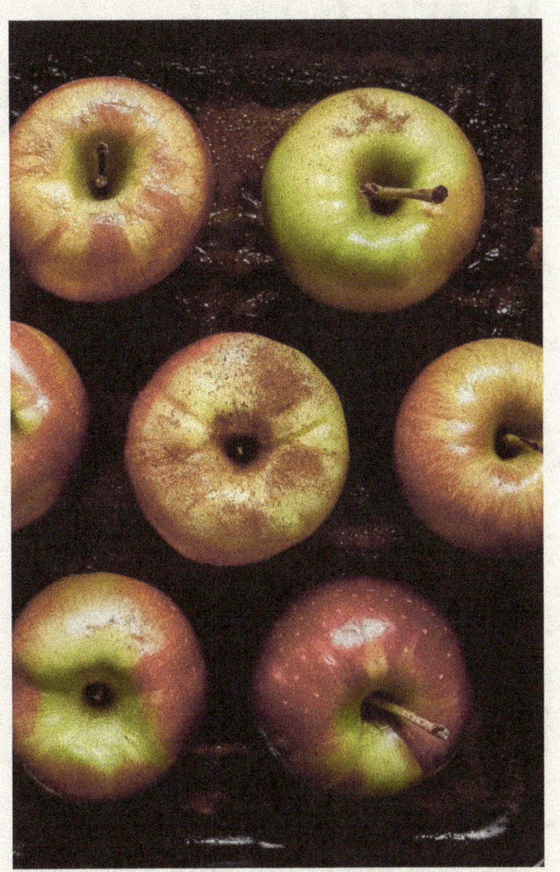

Instructions

- Preheat your oven to 375°F (190°C).
- Wash the apples and remove the cores, leaving the bottoms intact to hold the filling.
- Place the cored apples in a baking dish.
- Sprinkle ground cinnamon evenly over each apple.
- Bake for 25 minutes, or until the apples are tender.
- Serve warm as is or with a dollop of Greek yogurt or a scoop of vanilla ice cream, if desired.

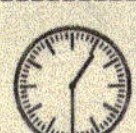 Preparation Time : 5 min

 Total Time : 30 min

Servings : 4

Nutritional Info

- Calories: 120 kcal
- Total Fat: 0.5g
- Carbohydrates: 31g
- Fiber: 5g
- Sugars: 24g
- Protein: 0.5g

BLUEBERRY AND LEMON SORBET

Ingredients

- 2 cups fresh blueberries
- 1/2 cup water
- 1/2 cup granulated sugar
- Zest and juice of 1 lemon

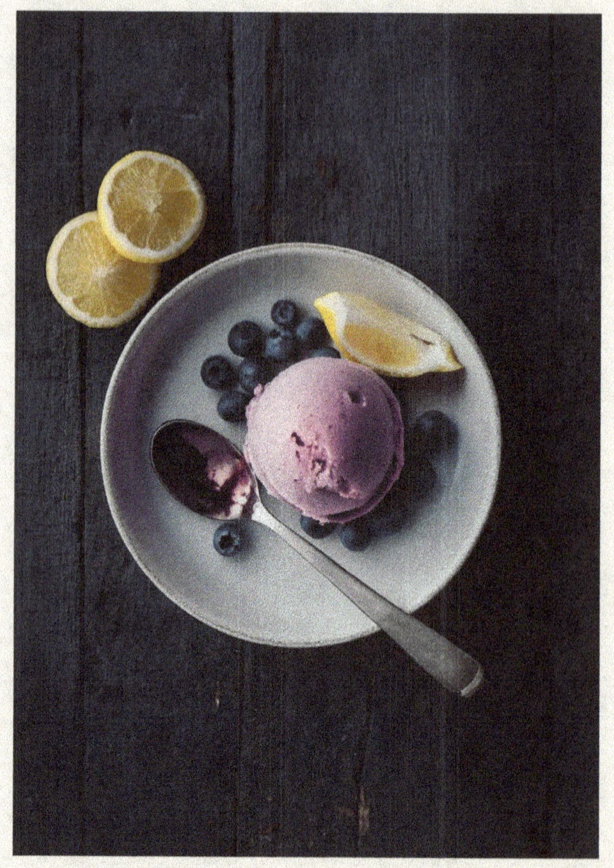

Instructions

- Combine Ingredients: In a saucepan, mix blueberries, water, and sugar. Heat on medium until sugar dissolves and blueberries soften (about 5 minutes).
- Blend: Pour mixture into a blender, add lemon zest and juice, blend until smooth.
- Strain (Optional): If desired, strain mixture through a sieve for smoother texture.
- Chill and Freeze: Cool mixture in the fridge for 2 hours. Pour into a shallow dish, freeze for 4-6 hours. Stir every hour.
- Serve: Scoop into bowls, garnish with blueberries or lemon zest. Enjoy!

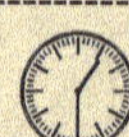 **Preparation Time : 10 min**

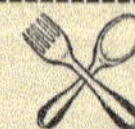 **Total Time : 15 min**

Servings : 4

Nutritional Info

- Calories: 80 kcal
- Fat: 0g
- Carbohydrates: 20g
- Fiber: 3g
- Sugars: 14g
- Protein: 1g

MANGO AND PINEAPPLE SALAD

Ingredients

- 1 ripe mango, peeled and diced
- 1 cup fresh pineapple chunks
- 1/4 cup red onion, finely chopped
- 1/4 cup fresh cilantro, chopped
- Juice of 1 lime
- Salt and pepper to taste

Instructions

- In a large mixing bowl, combine the diced mango, pineapple chunks, chopped red onion, and chopped cilantro.
- Squeeze the lime juice over the fruit mixture.
- Season with salt and pepper to taste.
- Gently toss the ingredients until everything is evenly coated with lime juice and seasoning.
- Serve immediately as a refreshing side dish or as a topping for grilled chicken or fish.

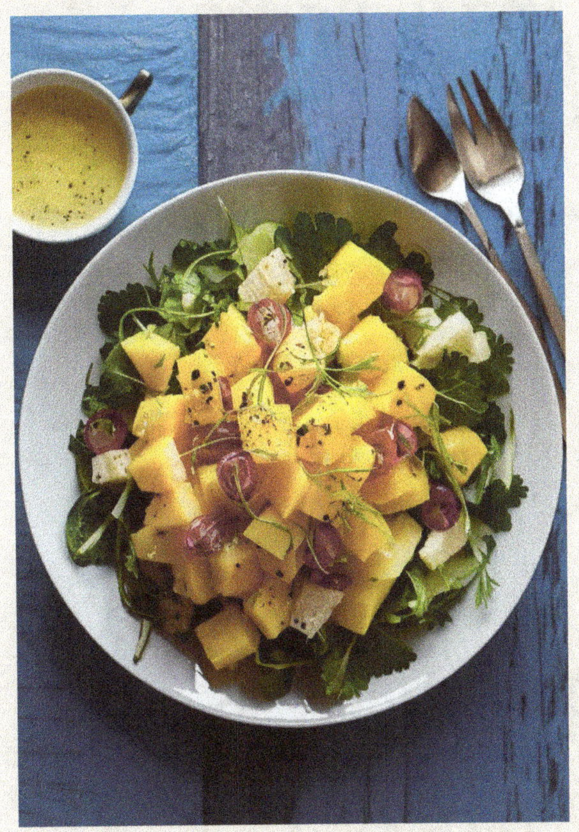

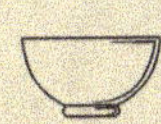 **Preparation Time : 10 min**

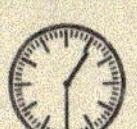 **Total Time : 0 min**

 **Servings : 4**

Nutritional Info

- Calories: 80 kcal
- Protein: 1g
- Carbohydrates: 21g
- Fat: 0g
- Fiber: 3g
- Sugar: 16g
- Sodium: 5mg

FROZEN YOGURT BARK WITH BERRIES

Ingredients

- 2 cups plain Greek yogurt
- 2 tablespoons honey or maple syrup
- 1 teaspoon vanilla extract
- 1 cup mixed berries (such as strawberries, blueberries, and raspberries)
- Optional: 2 tablespoons shredded coconut or chopped nuts for toppin

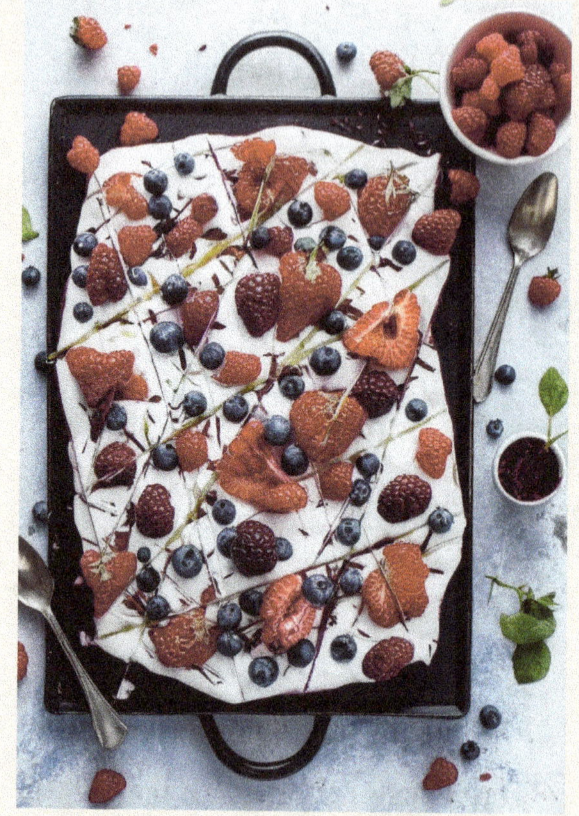

Instructions

- In a mixing bowl, combine the Greek yogurt, honey (or maple syrup), and vanilla extract. Stir until well combined.
- Line a baking sheet with parchment paper or a silicone baking mat.
- Pour the yogurt mixture onto the prepared baking sheet, spreading it evenly to about ¼ inch thickness.
- Scatter the mixed berries evenly over the yogurt mixture. Press them gently into the yogurt.
- If desired, sprinkle shredded coconut or chopped nuts over the top for added texture and flavor.
- Place the baking sheet in the freezer and let the yogurt bark freeze for at least 2 hours, or until completely firm.
- Once frozen, remove the baking sheet from the freezer and break the yogurt bark into pieces using your hands or a knife.
- Serve immediately as a refreshing snack or dessert. Store any leftovers in an airtight container in the freezer.

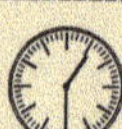 **Preparation Time : 10 min**

 **Total Time : 2hrs 10 min**

Servings : 6

Nutritional Info

- Calories: 110 kcal
- Total Fat: 2g
- Saturated Fat: 1g
- Cholesterol: 5mg
- Sodium: 25mg
- Total Carbohydrates: 14g

CHOCOLATE DIPPED STRAWBERRIES

Ingredients

- 1 pint of fresh strawberries, washed and dried
- 4 oz (about 120g) of dark chocolate chips or chopped dark chocolate (70% cocoa or higher)

Instructions

- Line a baking sheet with parchment paper.
- In a microwave-safe bowl, melt the dark chocolate chips in 30-second intervals, stirring in between, until smooth and fully melted.
- Hold each strawberry by the stem and dip it into the melted chocolate, swirling to coat it partially.
- Place the dipped strawberries onto the prepared baking sheet.
- Repeat with the remaining strawberries.
- Place the baking sheet in the refrigerator for about 15-20 minutes or until the chocolate sets.
- Once the chocolate has hardened, transfer the chocolate-dipped strawberries to a serving plate.
- Serve immediately as a delicious and healthy dessert option.

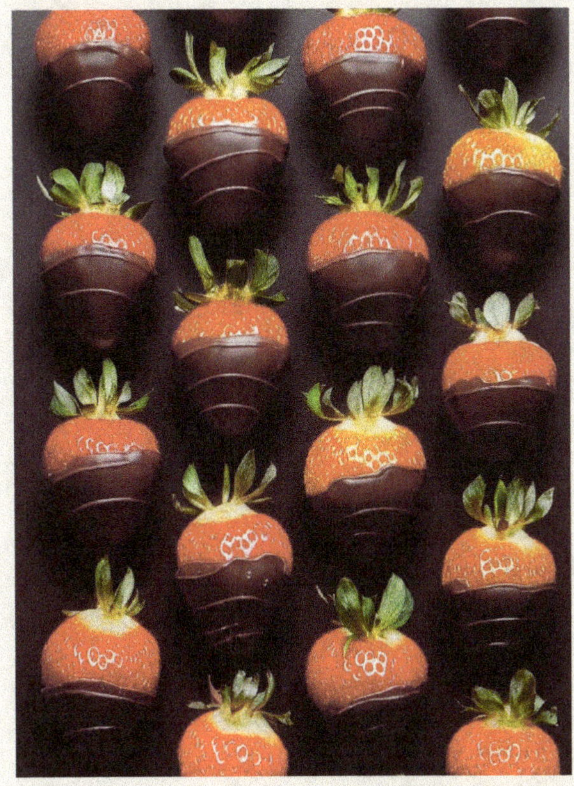

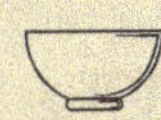 **Preparation Time : 10 min**

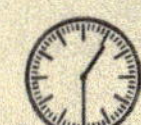 **Total Time : 15 min**

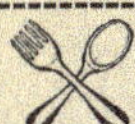 **Servings : 4**

Nutritional Info

- Calories: 120
- Total Fat: 7g
- Saturated Fat: 4g
- Cholesterol: 0mg
- Sodium: 5mg
- Total Carbohydrates: 15g

GRILLED PINEAPPLE WITH CINNAMON

Ingredients

- 1 ripe pineapple, peeled and cored
- 1 teaspoon ground cinnamon

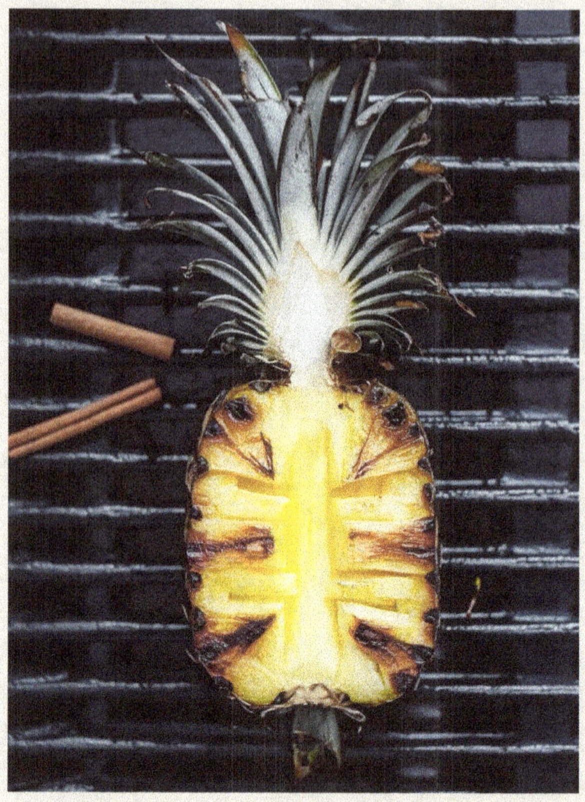

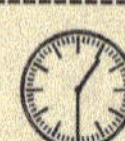 **Preparation Time : 10 min**

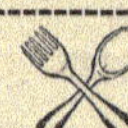 **Total Time : 5 min**

Servings : 2

Instructions

- Preheat your grill to medium-high heat.
- Slice the pineapple into rings or wedges, about 1/2 inch thick.
- Sprinkle both sides of the pineapple slices with ground cinnamon.
- Place the pineapple slices on the preheated grill.
- Grill for 3-4 minutes on each side, or until grill marks appear and the pineapple is heated through.
- Remove from the grill and serve hot.

Nutritional Info

- Calories: 90
- Total Fat: 0g
- Saturated Fat: 0g
- Cholesterol: 0mg
- Sodium: 0mg
- Total Carbohydrates: 23g

COCONUT MACAROONS

Ingredients

- 3 cups shredded coconut
- 3/4 cup sweetened condensed milk
- 2 large egg whites
- 1 teaspoon vanilla extract
- Pinch of salt

Instructions

- Preheat your oven to 325°F (160°C). Line a baking sheet with parchment paper.
- In a large bowl, combine the shredded coconut, sweetened condensed milk, vanilla extract, and salt. Mix well until evenly combined.
- In a separate bowl, beat the egg whites until stiff peaks form.
- Gently fold the beaten egg whites into the coconut mixture until fully incorporated.
- Using a spoon or cookie scoop, drop rounded tablespoons of the mixture onto the prepared baking sheet, spacing them about 1 inch apart.
- Bake in the preheated oven for 20-25 minutes, or until the macaroons are golden brown on the edges.
- Remove from the oven and let cool on the baking sheet for a few minutes before transferring to a wire rack to cool completely.

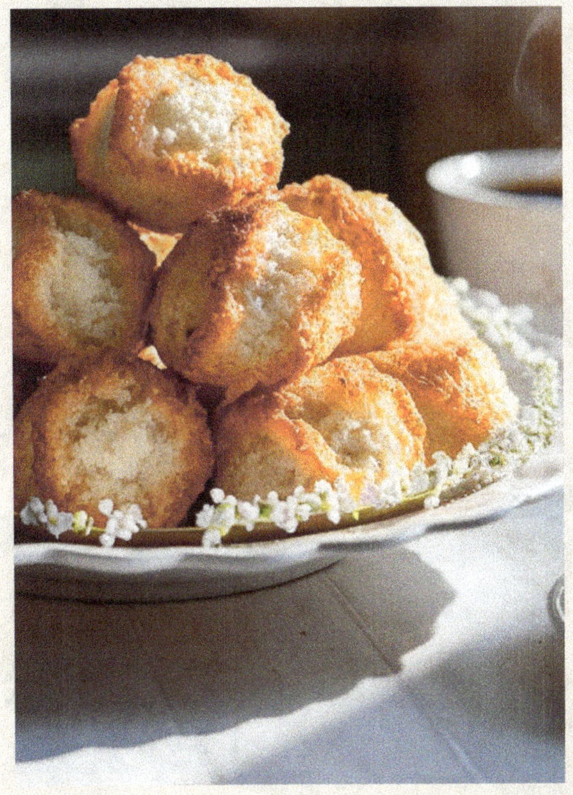

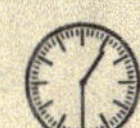 **Preparation Time : 10 min**

 **Total Time : 35 min**

Servings : 20 macaroons

Nutritional Info

- Calories: 120 kcal
- Total Fat: 7g
- Saturated Fat: 6g
- Trans Fat: 0g
- Cholesterol: 3mg
- Sodium: 60mg

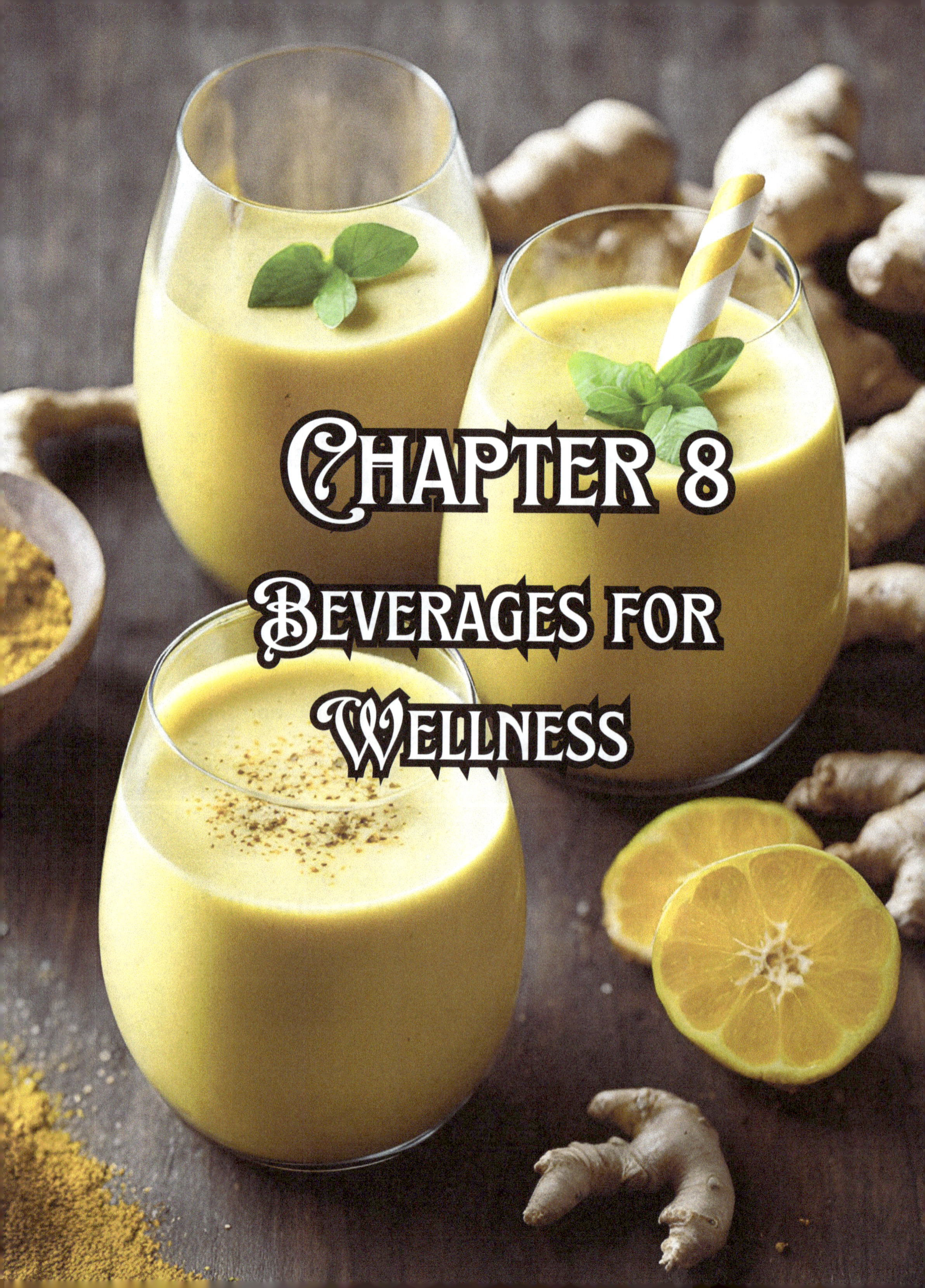
Chapter 8
Beverages for Wellness

WATERMELON COOLER

Ingredients

- 2 cups of diced seedless watermelon
- 1/2 cup of fresh lime juice
- 1 tablespoon of honey or agave syrup (optional)
- Ice cubes
- Fresh mint leaves for garnish (optional)

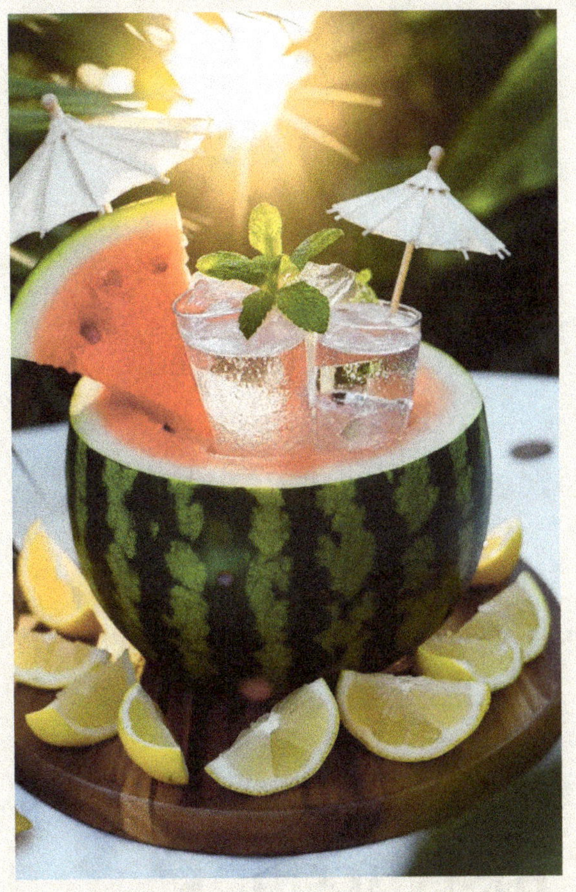

Instructions

- In a blender, combine the diced watermelon, lime juice, and honey (if using).
- Blend until smooth and well combined.
- Taste and adjust sweetness if necessary by adding more honey.
- Fill a glass with ice cubes.
- Pour the watermelon mixture over the ice cubes.
- Garnish with fresh mint leaves if desired.
- Serve immediately and enjoy!

🥣 **Preparation Time : 5 min**

🕐 **Total Time : 10 min**

🍴 **Servings : 1**

Nutritional Info

- Calories: 70 kcal
- Total Fat: 0 g
- Saturated Fat: 0 g
- Cholesterol: 0 mg
- Sodium: 2 mg
- Total Carbohydrates: 18 g

Ingredients

- 1 medium cucumber, thinly sliced
- 1/4 cup fresh mint leaves
- 1 lemon, thinly sliced
- 4 cups cold water
- Ice cubes (optional)

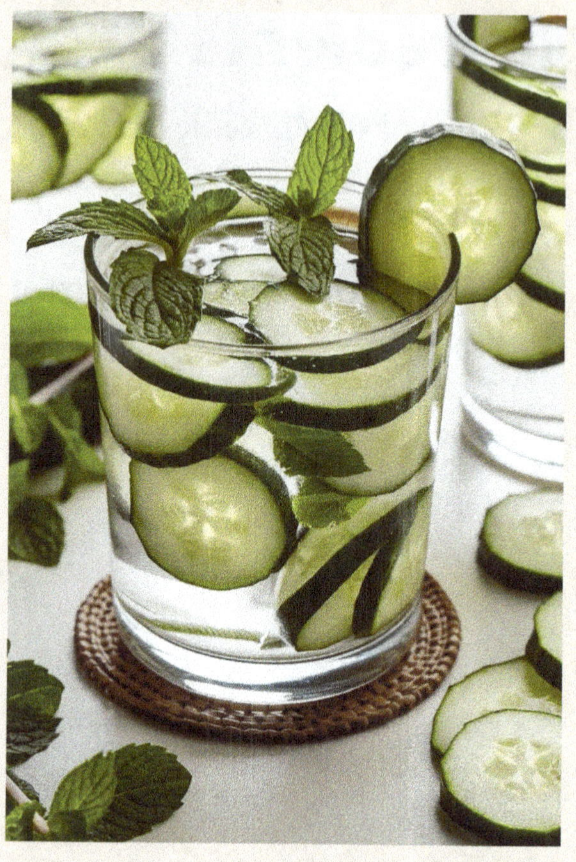

Instructions

- In a large pitcher, add the sliced cucumber, fresh mint leaves, and lemon slices.
- Pour cold water over the ingredients in the pitcher.
- Stir gently to combine.
- Refrigerate the cucumber mint water for at least 1 hour to allow the flavors to infuse.
- Serve chilled over ice cubes, if desired.

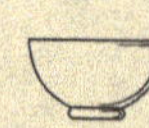 **Preparation Time : 5 min**

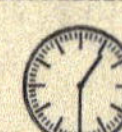 **Total Time : 5 min**

 **Servings : 4**

Nutritional Info

- Calories: 4
- Total Fat: 0g
- Cholesterol: 0mg
- Sodium: 2mg
- Total Carbohydrates: 1g
- Dietary Fiber: 0g

LEMON LIME INFUSION

Ingredients

- 1 lemon, thinly sliced
- 1 lime, thinly sliced
- Ice cubes (optional)
- Water

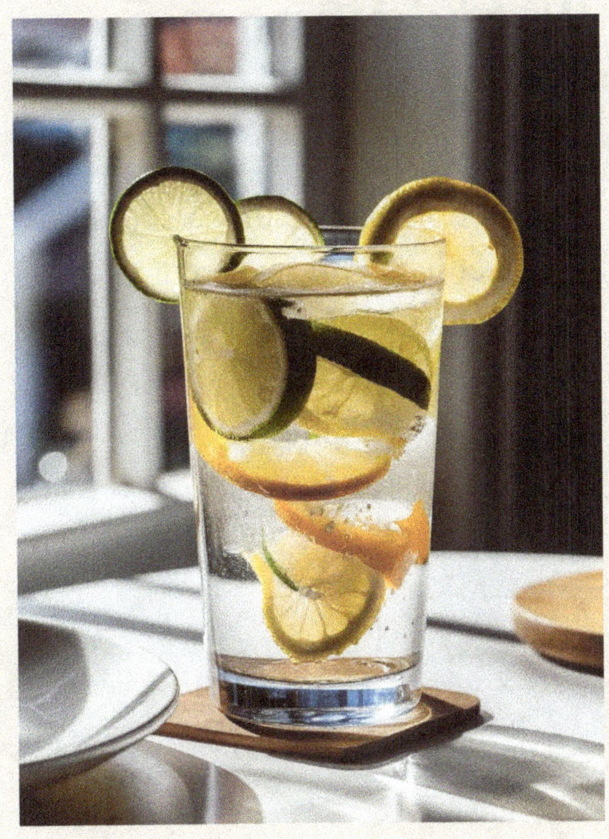

Instructions

- Place lemon and lime slices into a pitcher.
- Add ice cubes if desired.
- Fill the pitcher with water.
- Allow the water to infuse for at least 30 minutes before serving.
- Serve chilled and enjoy!

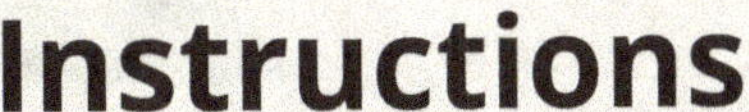 **Preparation Time : 5 min**

Total Time : 5 min

Servings : 1

Nutritional Info

- Calories: 0
- Carbohydrates: 0g
- Fat: 0g
- Protein: 0g

TROPICAL FRUIT SMOOTHIE

Ingredients

- 1/2 cup frozen pineapple chunks
- 1/2 cup frozen mango chunks
- 1/2 cup frozen banana slices
- 1/2 cup coconut water
- 1/4 cup Greek yogurt
- 1 tablespoon honey (optional)
- Juice of 1/2 lime

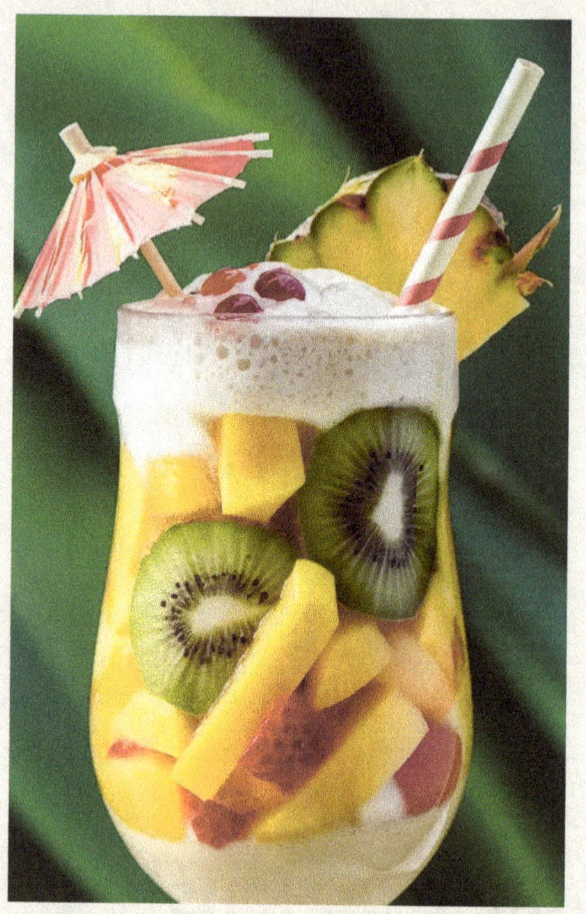

Instructions

- Place the frozen pineapple, mango, and banana chunks in a blender.
- Add the coconut water, Greek yogurt, honey (if using), and lime juice.
- Blend on high speed until smooth and creamy, adding more coconut water if necessary to reach your desired consistency.
- Pour into a glass and serve immediately.

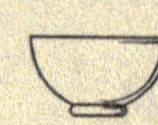 **Preparation Time : 5 min**

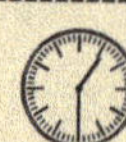 **Total Time : 5 min**

 **Servings : 1**

Nutritional Info

- Calories: 150
- Protein: 3g
- Carbohydrates: 35g
- Fat: 1g
- Fiber: 5g
- Sugar: 25g

BERRY PROTEIN SHAKE

Ingredients

- 1/2 cup mixed berries (strawberries, blueberries, raspberries)
- 1/2 cup unsweetened almond milk
- 1 scoop (about 30g) vanilla protein powder
- 1/4 cup plain Greek yogurt
- 1/2 banana, frozen
- 1/2 cup ice cubes

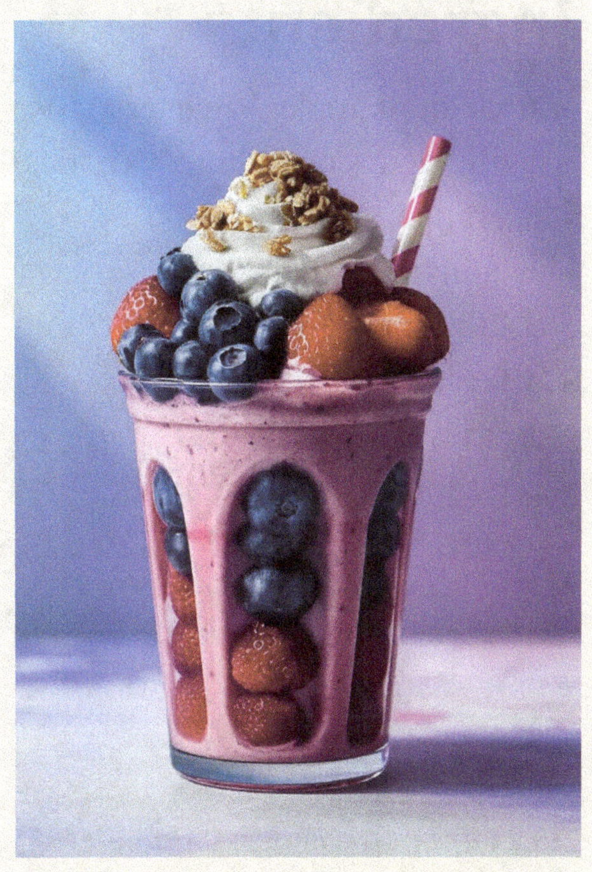

Instructions

- Add all ingredients to a blender.
- Blend on high speed until smooth and creamy, about 1-2 minutes.
- If the shake is too thick, add more almond milk, a little at a time, until desired consistency is reached.
- Pour into a glass and enjoy immediately!

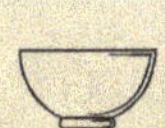 **Preparation Time : 5 min**

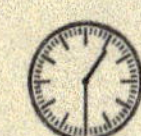 **Total Time : 5 min**

 **Servings : 1**

Nutritional Info

- Calories: 200 kcal
- Protein: 20g
- Carbohydrates: 25g
- Fat: 2g
- Fiber: 5g

SPICED APPLE CIDER

Ingredients

- 6 medium apples, quartered (use a mix of sweet and tart varieties)
- 1 orange, sliced
- 3 cinnamon sticks
- 1 tablespoon whole cloves
- 1 tablespoon whole allspice berries
- 1 teaspoon ground nutmeg
- 8 cups water

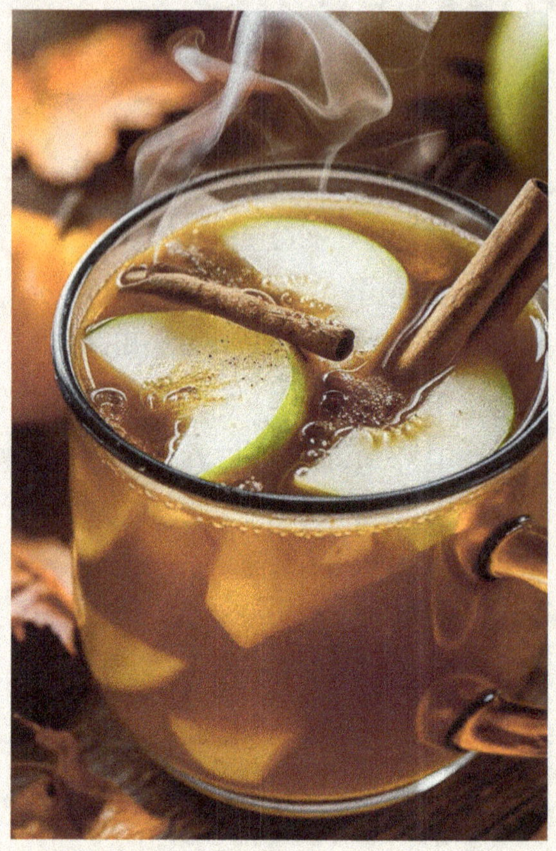

Instructions

- In a large pot, combine the quartered apples, orange slices, cinnamon sticks, whole cloves, whole allspice berries, ground nutmeg, and water.
- Bring the mixture to a boil over medium-high heat.
- Once boiling, reduce the heat to low and let the cider simmer for 30 minutes, uncovered, stirring occasionally.
- After 30 minutes, remove the pot from the heat and let it cool slightly.
- Using a fine mesh strainer or cheesecloth, strain the cider into a pitcher or another container to remove the solids.
- Serve the spiced apple cider warm, or refrigerate it for a few hours to serve chilled.
- Optionally, garnish each serving with a cinnamon stick or a slice of fresh apple.

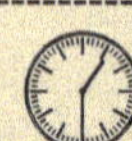 **Preparation Time : 5 min**

 **Total Time : 35 min**

Servings : 4

Nutritional Info

- Calories: 60
- Total Fat: 0g
- Saturated Fat: 0g
- Cholesterol: 0mg
- Sodium: 5mg
- Total Carbohydrates: 16g

MATCHA GREEN TEA LATTE

Ingredients

- 1 teaspoon matcha green tea powder
- 1/4 cup hot water (not boiling)
- 3/4 cup unsweetened almond milk (or any milk of choice)
- 1-2 teaspoons honey or sweetener of choice (optional)

Instructions

- Prepare Matcha: Sift 1 teaspoon of matcha green tea powder into a mug to avoid clumps.
- Add Water: Pour 1/4 cup of hot water (not boiling) into the mug with the matcha powder. Whisk vigorously using a bamboo whisk or a small regular whisk until the matcha is fully dissolved and frothy.
- Heat Milk: In a small saucepan, heat 3/4 cup of unsweetened almond milk over medium heat until it is warm but not boiling. You can also heat the milk in the microwave for about 1-2 minutes.
- Combine: Pour the heated milk into the mug with the matcha mixture. Stir to combine.
- Sweeten (Optional): If desired, add 1-2 teaspoons of honey or your preferred sweetener and stir until dissolved.
- Serve: Enjoy your Matcha Green Tea Latte immediately while warm.

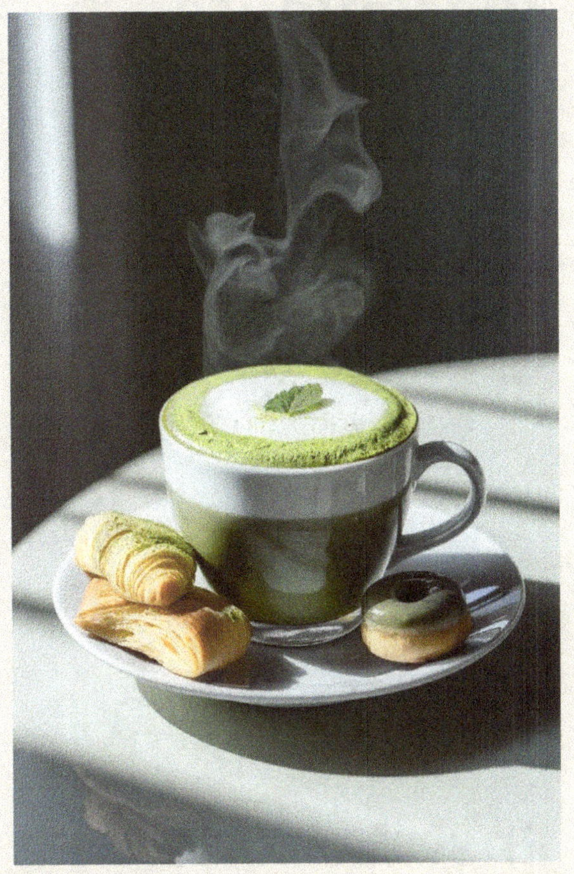

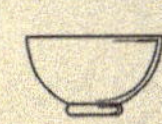 **Preparation Time : 5 min**

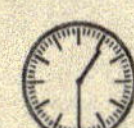 **Total Time : 10 min**

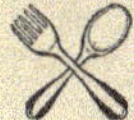 **Servings : 1**

Nutritional Info

- Calories: 40 (without sweetener)
- Protein: 1g
- Fat: 3g
- Carbohydrates: 2g
- Fiber: 1g
- Sugar: 0g (without sweetener)

GREEN DETOX SMOOTHIE

Ingredients

- 1 cup spinach, washed
- 1/2 cup kale, washed and stems removed
- 1/2 ripe avocado, peeled and pitted
- 1/2 banana, peeled
- 1/2 cup cucumber, peeled and chopped
- 1/2 cup unsweetened almond milk (or any milk of choice)
- Juice of 1/2 lemon
- 1 teaspoon grated ginger

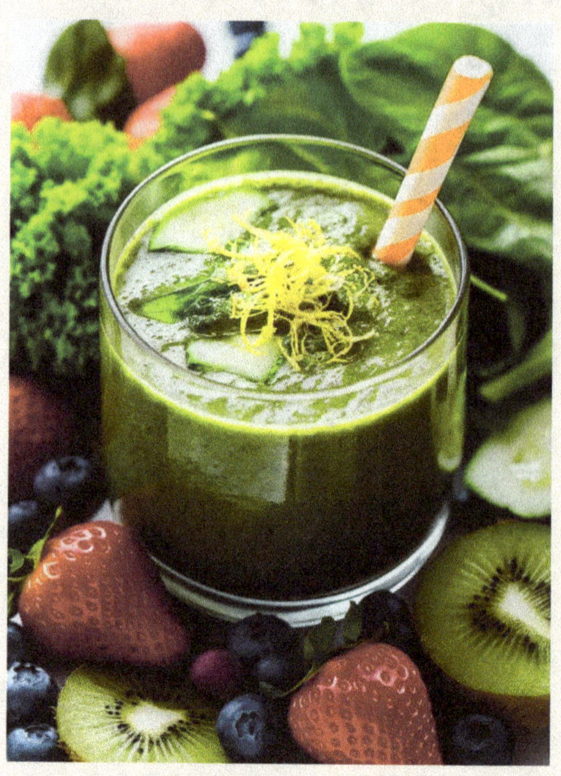

Instructions

- Place all the ingredients into a blender.
- Blend on high speed until smooth and creamy.
- If the smoothie is too thick, add more almond milk to reach your desired consistency.
- Taste and adjust sweetness by adding more banana if needed.
- Pour into a glass and enjoy immediately.

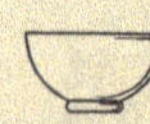 **Preparation Time : 5 min**

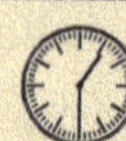 **Total Time : 5 min**

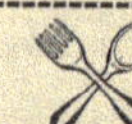 **Servings : 1**

Nutritional Info

- Calories: 150 kcal
- Protein: 5g
- Carbohydrates: 25g
- Fat: 3g
- Fiber: 8g

HERBAL ICED TEA

Ingredients

- 1 herbal tea bag (such as chamomile, peppermint, or hibiscus)
- 1 cup water
- Ice cubes
- Optional: sweetener of your choice (honey, stevia, agave syrup)

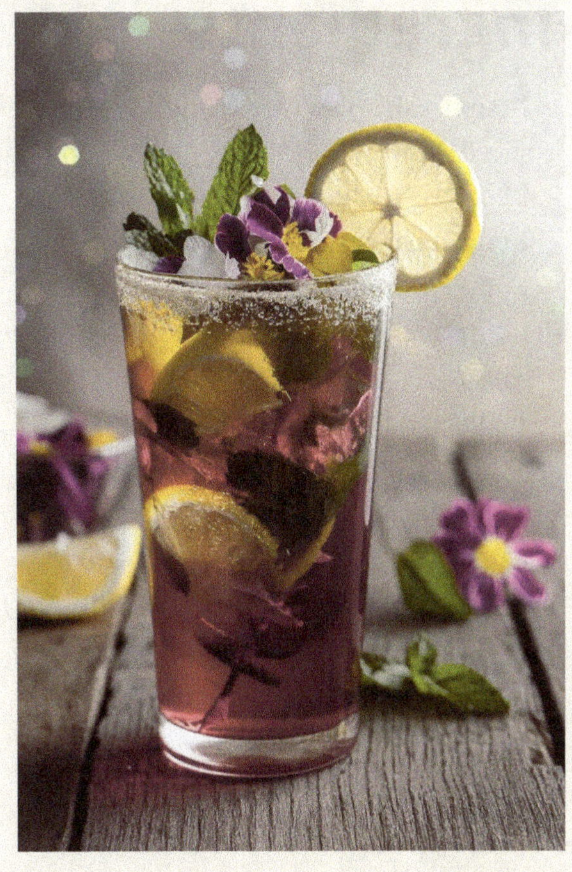

Instructions

- Boil 1 cup of water in a kettle or saucepan.
- Place the herbal tea bag in a heat-proof glass or mug.
- Pour the boiling water over the tea bag.
- Let the tea steep for 3-5 minutes, depending on your desired strength.
- Remove the tea bag and discard it.
- Allow the brewed tea to cool to room temperature.
- Once cooled, transfer the tea to a glass filled with ice cubes.
- Optionally, sweeten the tea with your preferred sweetener, stirring until dissolved.
- Garnish with a slice of lemon, a sprig of mint, or a slice of cucumber, if desired.
- Serve immediately and enjoy your refreshing Herbal Iced Tea!

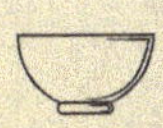 **Preparation Time : 5 min**

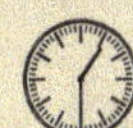 **Total Time : 5 min**

 **Servings : 1**

Nutritional Info

- Calories: 0 kcal
- Carbohydrates: 0 g
- Protein: 0 g
- Fat: 0 g
- Fiber: 0 g

BERRY LEMONADE

Ingredients

- 1 cup fresh strawberries, hulled and sliced
- 1 cup fresh blueberries
- 1 cup fresh raspberries
- 1 cup fresh blackberries
- 1 cup fresh lemon juice (about 4-6 lemons)
- 4 cups cold water
- 1-2 tablespoons honey or a natural sweetener (optional)
- Ice cubes
- Fresh mint leaves for garnish (optional)

Instructions

- Wash the strawberries, blueberries, raspberries, and blackberries thoroughly.
- Hull and slice the strawberries.
- Place the strawberries, blueberries, raspberries, and blackberries in a blender.
- Blend until smooth.
- Pour the blended berry mixture through a fine mesh sieve or cheesecloth into a large pitcher to remove seeds and pulp. Use a spoon to press the mixture through the sieve if needed.
- Add the freshly squeezed lemon juice to the pitcher.
- Pour in the cold water and stir well.
- If desired, add honey or your preferred natural sweetener to the pitcher and stir until dissolved.
- Fill glasses with ice cubes.
- Pour the berry lemonade over the ice.
- Garnish with fresh mint leaves if desired.
- Serve immediately and enjoy your refreshing berry lemonade!

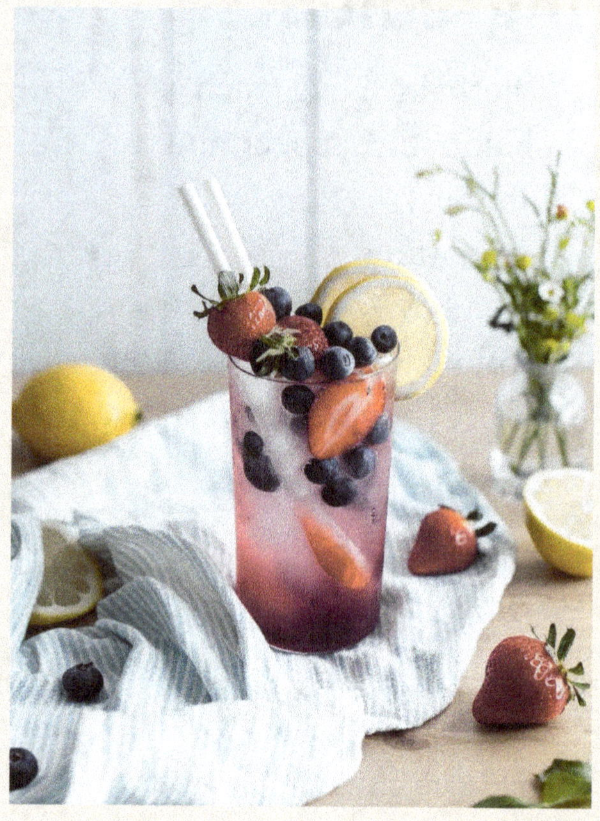

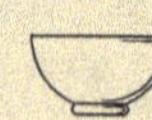
Preparation Time : 15 min

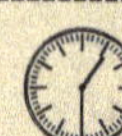
Total Time : 15 min

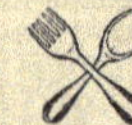
Servings : 4

Nutritional Info

- Calories: 50
- Protein: 1g
- Carbohydrates: 13g
- Dietary Fiber: 4g
- Sugars: 9g
- Fat: 0g

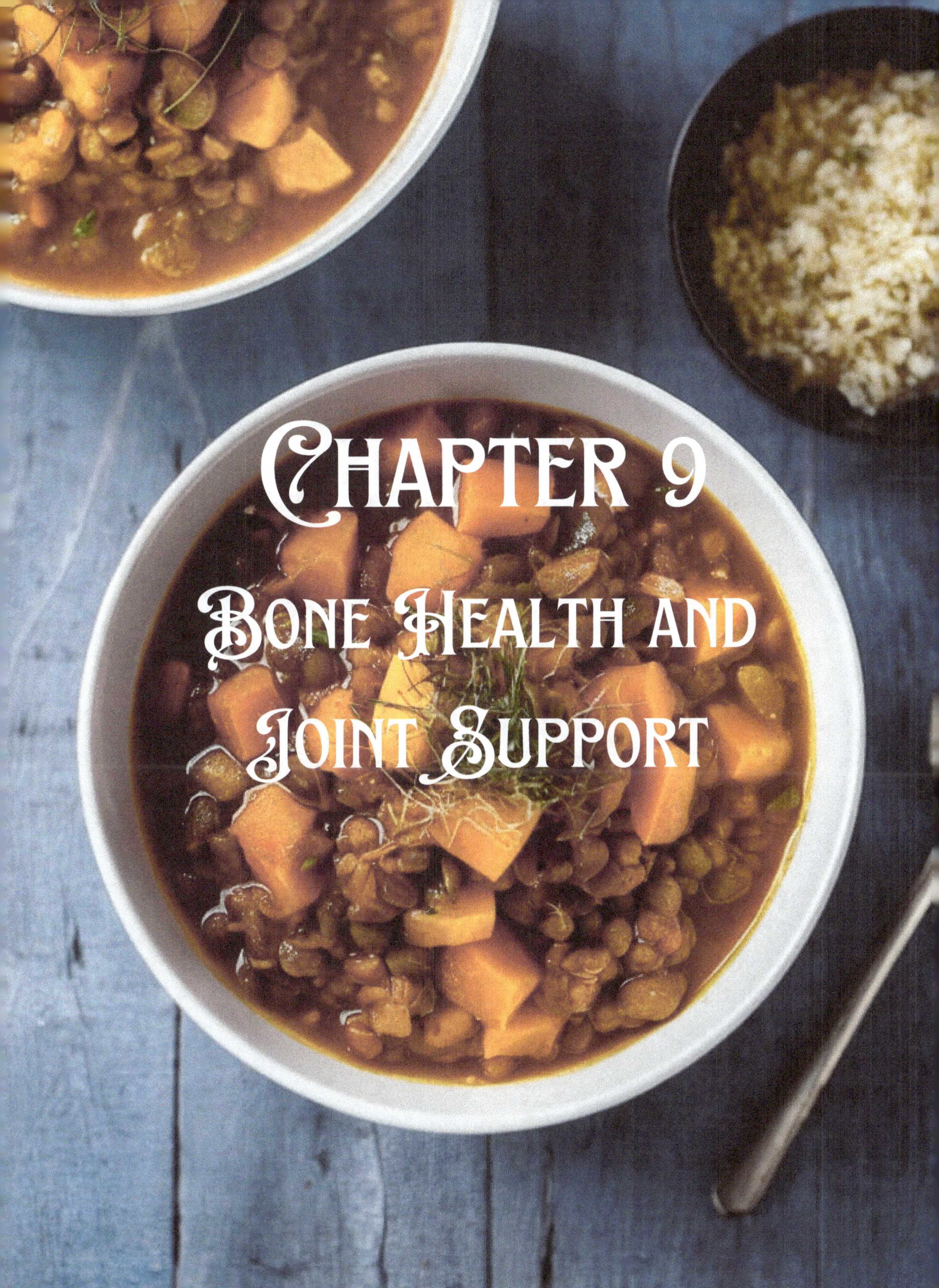

Chapter 9
Bone Health and Joint Support

SARDINE AND ARUGULA SALAD

Ingredients

- 2 cans of sardines, drained
- 4 cups fresh arugula
- 1 cup cherry tomatoes, halved
- 1/4 red onion, thinly sliced
- 1/4 cup Kalamata olives, pitted
- 2 tablespoons extra virgin olive oil
- 1 tablespoon balsamic vinegar
- Salt and pepper to taste

Instructions

- In a large bowl, combine the arugula, cherry tomatoes, red onion, and Kalamata olives.
- Add the drained sardines on top.
- In a small bowl, whisk together the olive oil, balsamic vinegar, salt, and pepper.
- Drizzle the dressing over the salad and gently toss to combine.
- Serve immediately.

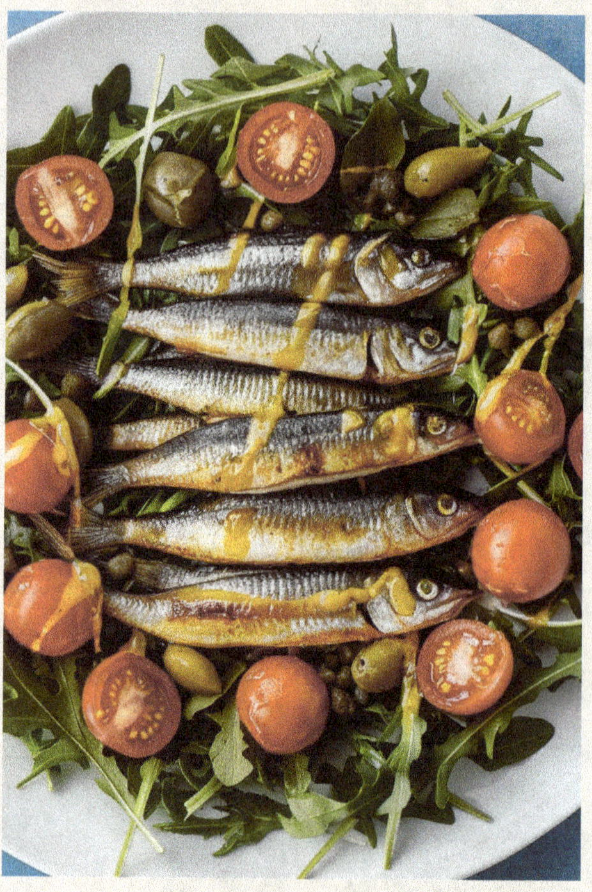

Preparation Time : 10 min

Total Time : 10 min

Servings : 2

Nutritional Info

- Calories: 320 kcal
- Protein: 24g
- Carbohydrates: 7g
- Fat: 22g
- Fiber: 2g

ALMOND-CRUSTED CHICKEN TENDERS

Ingredients

- 1 lb chicken tenders
- 1 cup almond flour
- 2 eggs, beaten
- 1 tsp garlic powder
- 1 tsp paprika
- Salt and pepper to taste
- Cooking spray or olive oil

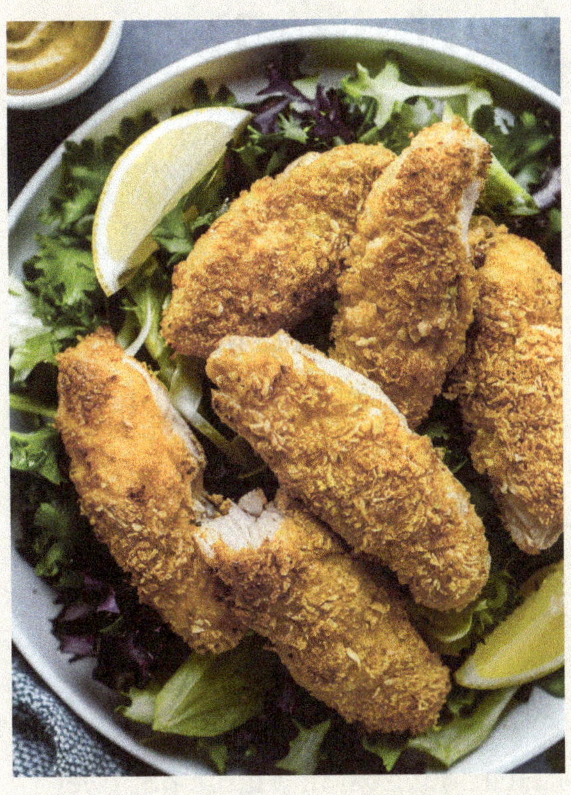

Instructions

- Preheat your oven to 400°F (200°C).
- In a shallow dish, mix almond flour, garlic powder, paprika, salt, and pepper.
- Dip each chicken tender into the beaten eggs, then coat with the almond flour mixture, pressing gently to adhere.
- Place the coated tenders on a baking sheet lined with parchment paper or aluminum foil.
- Lightly spray or drizzle with olive oil.
- Bake for 15-20 minutes or until the chicken is cooked through and the coating is golden brown and crispy.
- Serve hot with your favorite dipping sauce.

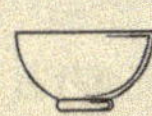 **Preparation Time : 10 min**

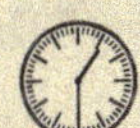 **Total Time : 25 min**

 **Servings : 4**

Nutritional Info

- Calories: 290 kcal
- Protein: 30g
- Fat: 16g
- Saturated Fat: 2g
- Trans Fat: 0g

BROCCOLI AND KALE SOUP

Ingredients

- 2 cups broccoli florets
- 1 cup chopped kale leaves
- 1 onion, diced
- 2 cloves garlic, minced
- 4 cups vegetable broth
- 1 tablespoon olive oil
- Salt and pepper to taste

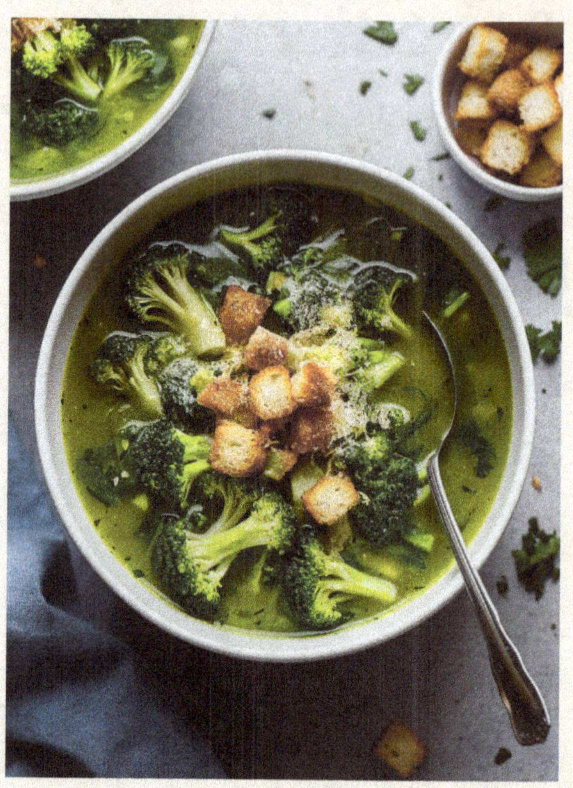

Instructions

- Heat olive oil in a large pot over medium heat. Add diced onion and minced garlic, sauté until fragrant.
- Add broccoli florets and chopped kale leaves to the pot. Cook for 5 minutes, stirring occasionally.
- Pour vegetable broth into the pot. Bring to a boil, then reduce heat and simmer for 15-20 minutes until vegetables are tender.
- Use an immersion blender or transfer soup to a blender to puree until smooth.
- Season with salt and pepper to taste. If desired, add red pepper flakes for heat.
- Serve hot, garnished with grated Parmesan if desired.

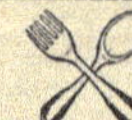 Preparation Time : 10 min

Total Time : 30 min

Servings : 4

Nutritional Info

- Calories: 120 kcal
- Protein: 4g
- Carbohydrates: 15g
- Fat: 6g
- Fiber: 5g

SESAME GINGER TOFU

Ingredients

- 1 block (14 oz) firm tofu, drained and pressed
- 2 tbsp soy sauce
- 1 tbsp sesame oil
- 1 tbsp rice vinegar
- 1 tbsp maple syrup or honey
- 2 cloves garlic, minced
- 1 tbsp freshly grated ginger or ginger paste
- 2 tbsp sesame seeds
- 2 green onions, thinly sliced
- 1 tbsp cornstarch
- 2 tbsp water

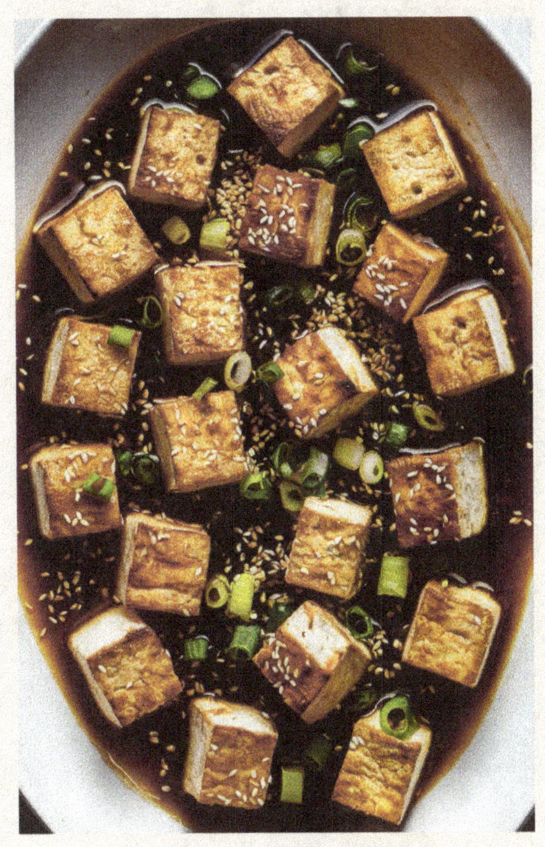

Instructions

- Cut tofu into cubes or slices.
- In a bowl, mix soy sauce, sesame oil, rice vinegar, maple syrup, minced garlic, grated ginger, and sesame seeds.
- Toss tofu in the marinade, coat evenly.
- Let it sit for 15-30 minutes.
- Mix cornstarch and water in a small bowl.
- Heat cooking oil in a pan over medium-high heat.
- Dip each tofu piece in the cornstarch mixture.
- Fry tofu until golden brown and crispy, about 3-4 minutes per side.
- Remove from pan and drain excess oil on paper towels.
- Garnish with sliced green onions and sesame seeds.
- Serve hot as a main dish or with rice and vegetables.

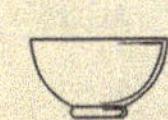 **Preparation Time : 15 min**

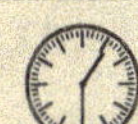 **Total Time : 25 min**

 **Servings : 4**

Nutritional Info

- Calories: 220 kcal
- Protein: 14g
- Carbohydrates: 10g
- Fat: 15g
- Fiber: 2g

CITRUS AND WALNUT SALAD

Ingredients

- 4 cups mixed salad greens
- 1 orange, segmented
- 1 grapefruit, segmented
- ½ cup walnuts, toasted
- ¼ cup crumbled feta cheese (optional)
- 2 tablespoons extra virgin olive oil
- 1 tablespoon balsamic vinegar
- Salt and pepper to taste

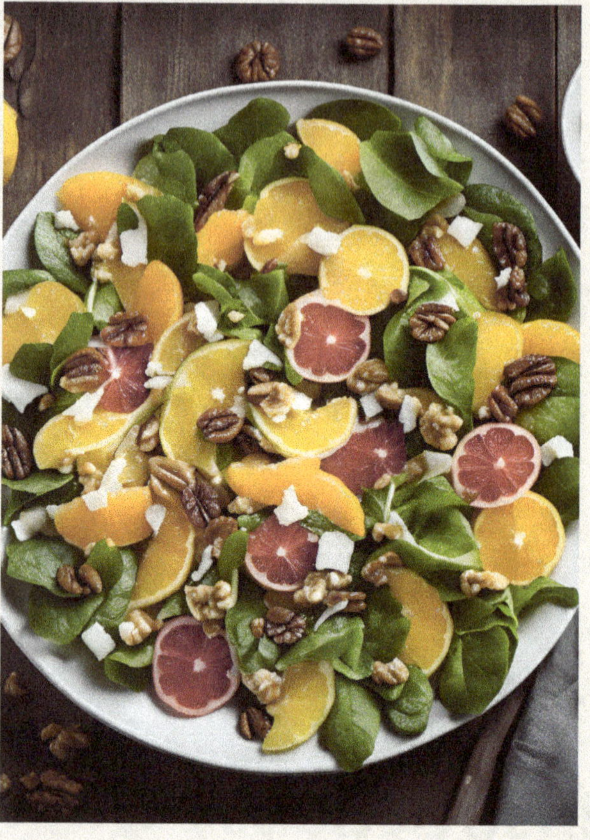

Instructions

- In a large bowl, combine the mixed salad greens, orange segments, and grapefruit segments.
- In a dry skillet over medium heat, toast the walnuts for 2-3 minutes until fragrant, then remove from heat and let them cool.
- Add the toasted walnuts to the bowl with the salad greens and citrus segments.
- If using, sprinkle the crumbled feta cheese over the salad.
- In a small bowl, whisk together the extra virgin olive oil and balsamic vinegar to make the dressing.
- Drizzle the dressing over the salad and toss gently to coat.
- Season with salt and pepper to taste.
- Serve immediately.

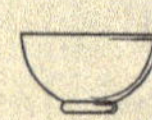 **Preparation Time : 10 min**

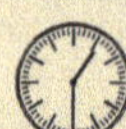 **Total Time : 15 min**

 **Servings : 4**

Nutritional Info

- Calories: 210 kcal
- Total Fat: 18g
- Saturated Fat: 2g
- Trans Fat: 0g
- Cholesterol: 0mg
- Sodium: 90mg

SPINACH AND RICOTTA STUFFED PORTOBELLOS

Ingredients

- 4 large portobello mushrooms
- 2 cups fresh spinach, chopped
- 1 cup ricotta cheese
- 1/2 cup grated Parmesan cheese
- 2 cloves garlic, minced
- Salt and pepper to taste
- Olive oil for drizzling

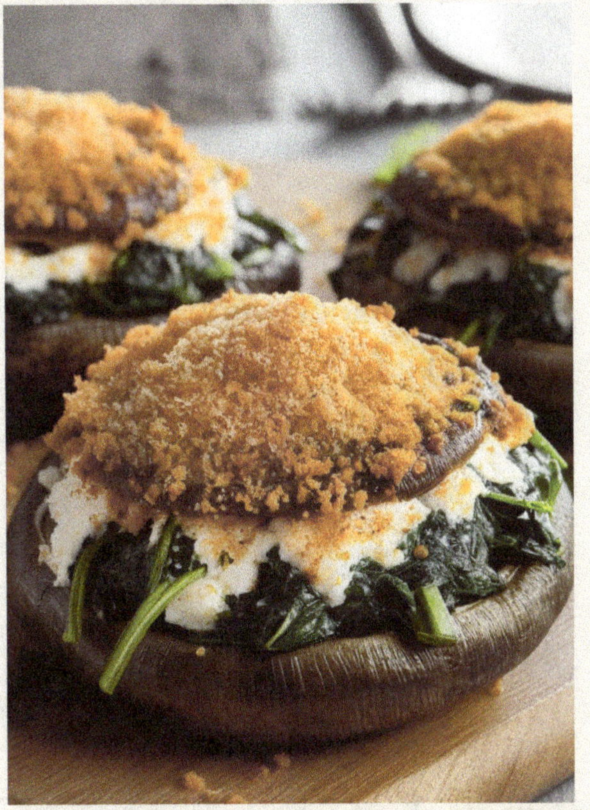

Instructions

- Preheat the oven to 375°F (190°C). Line a baking sheet with parchment paper.
- Clean the portobello mushrooms and remove the stems. Place them on the prepared baking sheet, gill side up.
- In a mixing bowl, combine chopped spinach, ricotta cheese, Parmesan cheese, minced garlic, salt, and pepper. Mix well.
- Spoon the spinach and ricotta mixture evenly into each portobello mushroom cap, filling them to the top.
- Drizzle olive oil over the stuffed mushrooms.
- Bake in the preheated oven for 20-25 minutes, or until the mushrooms are tender and the filling is golden brown.
- Garnish with fresh basil leaves if desired before serving.

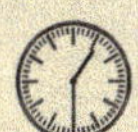 **Preparation Time : 15 min**

 **Total Time : 40 min**

Servings : 4

Nutritional Info

- Calories: 185 kcal
- Protein: 12g
- Carbohydrates: 8g
- Fat: 12g
- Fiber: 2g

MISO SOUP WITH SEAWEED

Ingredients

- 4 cups water
- 4 tablespoons miso paste
- 1 sheet nori seaweed, shredded
- 1 cup firm tofu, cubed
- 2 green onions, thinly sliced
- Optional: 1 tablespoon soy sauce or tamari for extra flavor

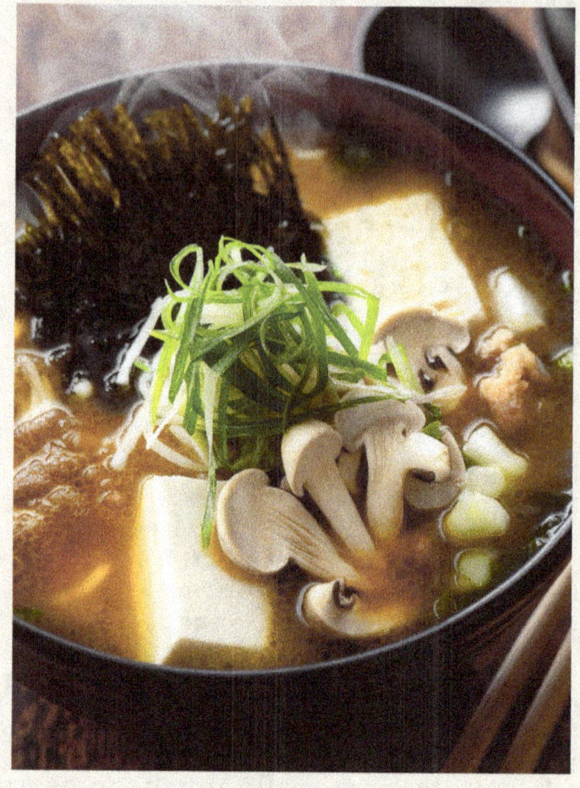

Instructions

- In a pot, bring water to a gentle boil.
- Reduce heat to low and whisk in miso paste until dissolved.
- Add shredded nori and tofu cubes, simmer for 5 minutes.
- Remove from heat and stir in green onions.
- Serve hot and enjoy!

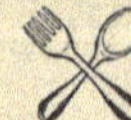 Preparation Time : 10 min

Total Time : 15 min

Servings : 4

Nutritional Info

- Calories: 90
- Total Fat: 4g
- Saturated Fat: 0.5g
- Trans Fat: 0g
- Cholesterol: 0mg

CALCIUM-RICH SMOOTHIE

Ingredients

- 1 cup kale leaves, stemmed
- 1 ripe banana
- 1/2 cup plain Greek yogurt
- 1/2 cup almond milk
- 1 tablespoon almond butter
- 1 tablespoon honey
- Ice cubes (optional)

Instructions

- Place all ingredients into a blender.
- Blend until smooth and creamy.
- If desired, add ice cubes and blend again until desired consistency is reached.
- Pour into glasses and serve immediately.

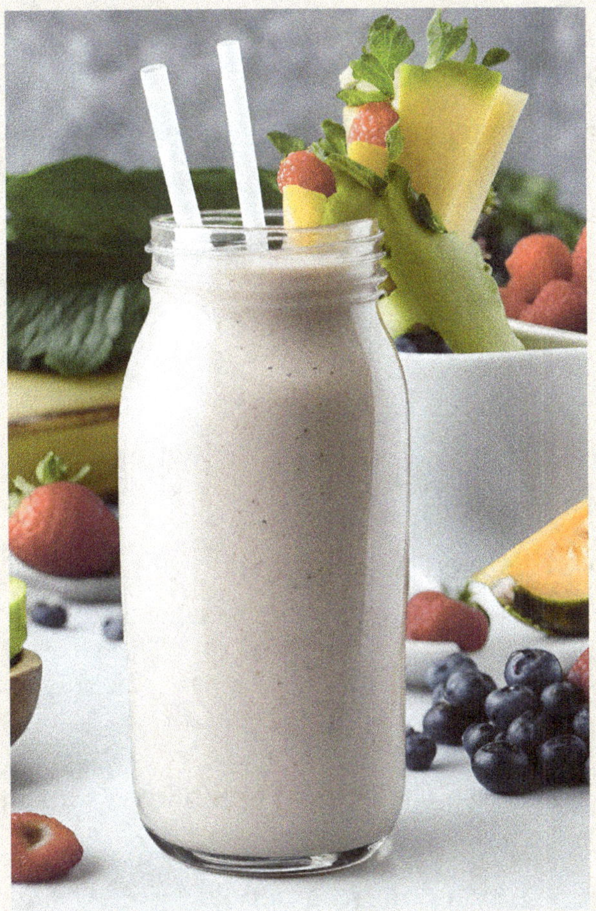

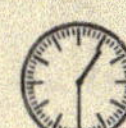 **Preparation Time : 5 min**

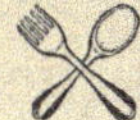 **Total Time : 5 min**

Servings : 2

Nutritional Info

- Calories: 180
- Protein: 9g
- Fat: 5g
- Carbohydrates: 30g
- Calcium: 25%

Ingredients

- Large collard green leaves
- Hummus
- Sliced avocado
- Sliced cucumber
- Shredded carrots
- Sliced bell peppers
- Cooked quinoa or brown rice (optional)
- Sliced tofu or grilled chicken (optional)

Instructions

- Wash the collard green leaves and pat them dry.
- Lay a collard green leaf flat on a clean surface.
- Spread a layer of hummus evenly across the leaf, leaving about an inch of space around the edges.
- Layer on sliced avocado, cucumber, shredded carrots, and bell peppers, along with any optional ingredients like quinoa or tofu/chicken.
- Carefully roll up the collard green leaf, tucking in the sides as you go, to form a wrap.
- Secure the wrap with toothpicks if needed.
- Slice the wrap in half diagonally.
- Serve immediately with your favorite sauce or dressing for dipping.

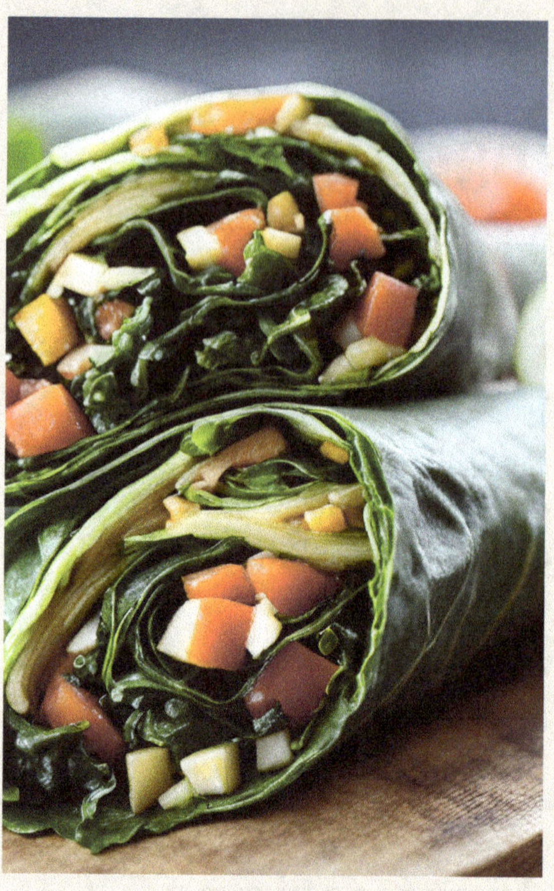

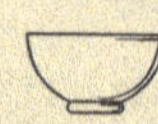 **Preparation Time : 15 min**

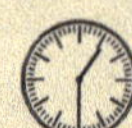 **Total Time : 15 min**

 **Servings : 4**

Nutritional Info

- Calories: Approximately 150-200 calories
- Protein: 5-10 grams
- Fat: 8-12 grams
- Carbohydrates: 15-20 grams
- Fiber: 5-8 grams

ORANGE AND ALMOND SALAD

Ingredients

- 2 large oranges, peeled and sliced
- 1/4 cup sliced almonds
- 4 cups mixed salad greens
- 1 tablespoon olive oil
- 1 tablespoon balsamic vinegar
- Salt and pepper to taste

Instructions

- In a dry skillet, toast the sliced almonds over medium heat until golden brown and fragrant, about 3-4 minutes. Remove from heat and set aside.
- In a large bowl, combine the mixed salad greens with the sliced oranges.
- In a small bowl, whisk together the olive oil and balsamic vinegar to make the dressing.
- Drizzle the dressing over the salad and toss gently to coat.
- Sprinkle the toasted almonds over the top of the salad.
- Season with salt and pepper to taste.
- Serve immediately and enjoy!

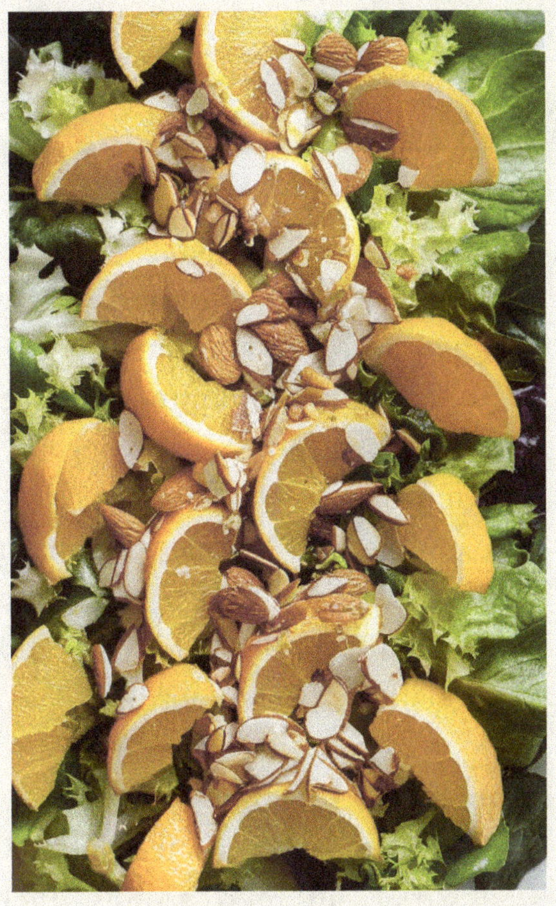

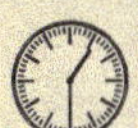
Preparation Time : 10 min

Total Time : 10 min

Servings : 4

Nutritional Info

- Calories: 120 kcal
- Total Fat: 8g
- Saturated Fat: 1g
- Trans Fat: 0g
- Cholesterol: 0mg
- Sodium: 80mg

How to Plan GERD-Friendly Meals

Understand Your Triggers:
- Tip: Keep a food diary to track what you eat and how it affects your GERD symptoms. Identify and avoid foods that trigger your symptoms.
- Example: If you notice that tomatoes or citrus fruits cause heartburn, eliminate or reduce these items from your diet.

Balance Your Plate:
- Tip: Aim for a balanced meal with a variety of food groups. Include lean proteins, whole grains, non-citrus fruits, and plenty of vegetables.
- Example: A balanced meal could include grilled chicken breast, quinoa, steamed broccoli, and a side of sliced apples.

Portion Control:
- Tip: Eating smaller, more frequent meals can help prevent overeating and reduce stomach pressure, which can minimize acid reflux.
- Example: Instead of three large meals, have five to six smaller meals throughout the day.

Choose Cooking Methods Wisely:
- Tip: Opt for baking, grilling, steaming, or broiling instead of frying foods, which can increase fat content and trigger GERD symptoms.
- Example: Bake fish with herbs and lemon instead of frying it.

Plan Ahead:
- Tip: Prepare meals and snacks in advance to ensure you always have GERD-friendly options available, especially on busy days.
- Example: Cook a batch of quinoa and grilled chicken at the beginning of the week and use them in salads, bowls, and wraps.

Incorporate High-Fiber Foods:
- Tip: Fiber aids digestion and can help prevent GERD symptoms by making you feel full and reducing the urge to overeat.
- Example: Include foods like oatmeal, whole grains, vegetables, fruits, and legumes in your meals.

Include Lean Proteins:

- Tip: Lean proteins are less likely to trigger GERD symptoms compared to high-fat meats.
- Example: Opt for skinless poultry, fish, tofu, and legumes over fatty cuts of meat.

Avoid Eating Before Bedtime:

- Tip: Finish eating at least 2-3 hours before lying down to prevent nighttime GERD symptoms.
- Example: If you go to bed at 10 PM, aim to have your last meal by 7 PM.

Stay Upright After Meals:

- Tip: Remain upright for at least 2-3 hours after eating to help food digest and prevent acid reflux.
- Example: After dinner, take a walk or stay seated instead of lying down.

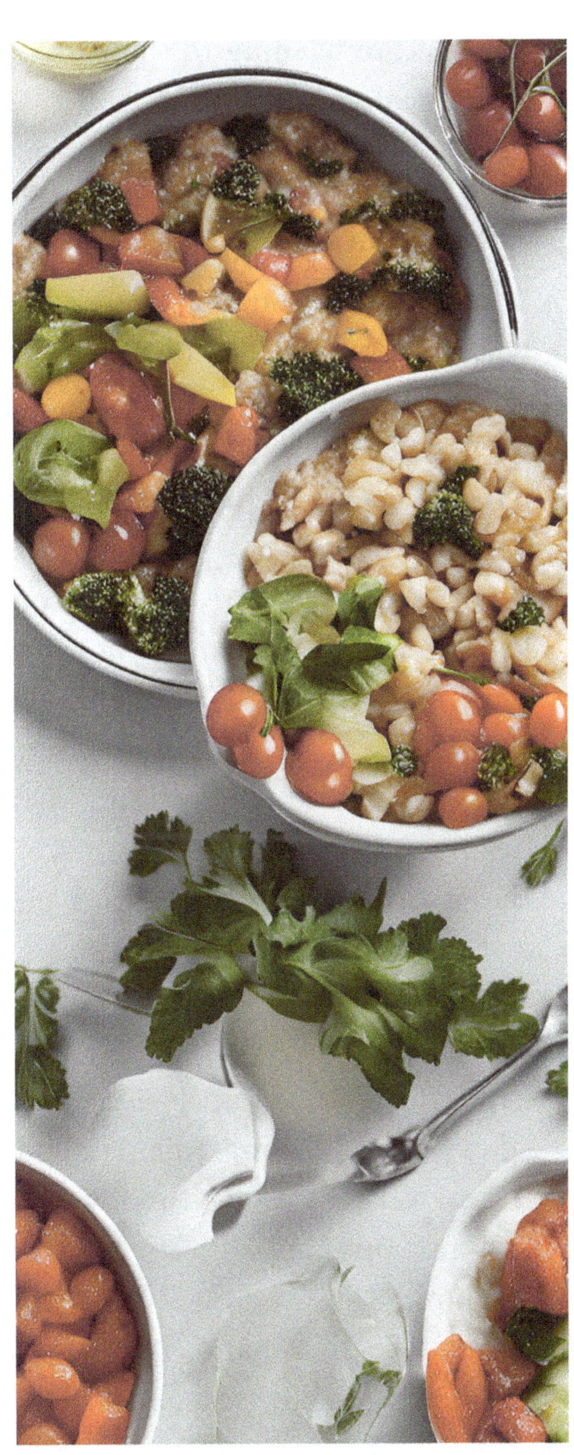

Grocery Shopping Tips for a GERD-Friendly Diet

Plan Your Meals and Make a List:
- Tip: Before heading to the store, plan your meals for the week and make a detailed grocery list to ensure you buy GERD-friendly foods.
- Example: List out ingredients for balanced meals such as lean proteins, whole grains, vegetables, and non-citrus fruits.

Shop the Perimeter of the Store:
- Tip: Focus on the perimeter of the grocery store where fresh produce, lean meats, dairy, and whole grains are typically located.
- Example: Spend most of your time in the produce section, meat department, and dairy aisle, avoiding the processed foods in the middle aisles.

Read Food Labels:
- Tip: Check food labels for high-fat, spicy, or acidic ingredients that can trigger GERD. Look for low-fat and low-acid options.
- Example: Choose low-fat yogurt over full-fat versions and opt for low-sodium, non-spicy seasoning blends.

Stock Up on Whole Grains:
- Tip: Whole grains are a great source of fiber and can help with digestion.
- Example: Buy **oatmeal,** brown rice, quinoa, whole wheat bread, and whole grain pasta.

Choose Fresh Fruits and Vegetables:
- Tip: Opt for a variety of fresh, non-citrus fruits and vegetables to ensure a nutrient-rich diet.
- Example: Buy apples, bananas, melons, leafy greens, carrots, broccoli, and green beans.

Select Lean Proteins:
- Tip: Lean proteins are less likely to trigger GERD symptoms and are essential for a balanced diet.
- Example: Purchase skinless chicken breasts, turkey, fish, tofu, and legumes like lentils and beans.

Choose Mild Herbs and Spices:
- Tip: Select herbs and spices that add flavor without causing irritation.
- Example: Buy fresh or dried basil, parsley, thyme, ginger, and other mild herbs.

Pick Non-Caffeinated Beverages:
- Tip: Avoid caffeinated and acidic drinks, and choose GERD-friendly beverages instead.
- Example: Purchase herbal teas like chamomile and ginger tea, as well as non-citrus juices such as apple or pear juice.

Consider Frozen and Canned Options:
- Tip: Frozen and canned fruits and vegetables can be convenient and nutritious alternatives, as long as they are low in added sugars and sodium.
- Example: Buy frozen berries, peas, and carrots, and canned beans and tomatoes (without added salt or seasoning).

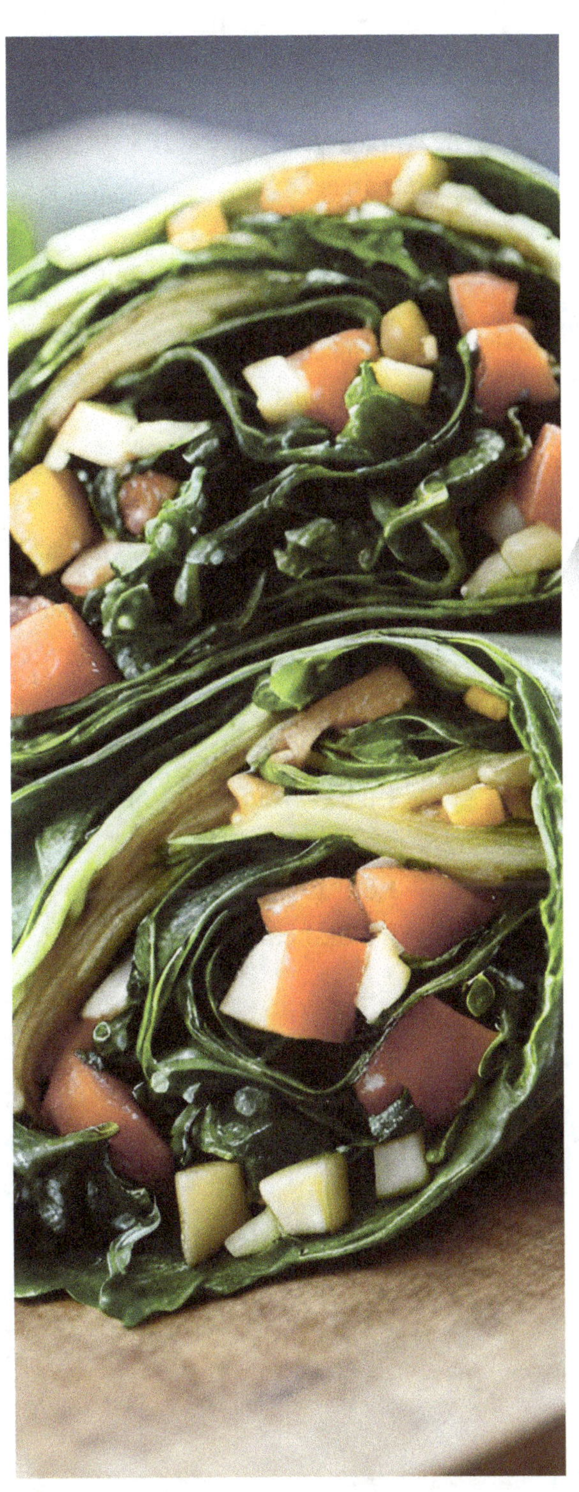

Sample Grocery List for GERD-Friendly Shopping

Produce

- Apples
- Bananas
- Melons
- Leafy greens (spinach, kale)
- Broccoli
- Carrots
- Green beans
- Cucumbers
- Sweet potatoes

Whole Grains

- Oatmeal
- Brown rice
- Quinoa
- Whole wheat bread
- Whole grain pasta

Proteins

- Chicken breasts
- Turkey
- Fish (salmon, tilapia)
- Tofu
- Lentils
- Black beans

Healthy Fats

- Avocados
- Almonds
- Chia seeds
- Olive oil

Dairy

- Skim milk
- Low-fat yogurt
- Low-fat cheese
- Almond milk

Frozen and Canned Goods

- Frozen berries
- Frozen peas
- Frozen carrots
- Canned black beans
- Canned tomatoes (no added salt)

GERD-Friendly Swaps

High-Fat Meats

- Swap: Fatty cuts of beef, pork, and lamb.
- For: Lean meats like skinless chicken breast, turkey, fish, and plant-based proteins such as tofu and legumes.
- Benefit: Reduces fat intake which can decrease the risk of acid reflux.

Full-Fat Dairy Products

- Swap: Whole milk, full-fat cheese, and regular ice cream.
- For: Skim milk, low-fat cheese, low-fat or non-fat yogurt, and dairy-free alternatives like almond milk or soy milk.
- Benefit: Lower fat content helps prevent GERD symptoms.

Spicy Foods

- Swap: Hot peppers, spicy sauces, and foods heavily seasoned with chili powder or hot sauce.
- For: Mild herbs and spices like basil, parsley, thyme, ginger, and turmeric.
- Benefit: Reduces irritation and inflammation of the esophagus.

Acidic Fruits and Juices

- Swap: Citrus fruits (oranges, lemons, grapefruits) and juices.
- For: Non-citrus fruits like bananas, melons, apples, pears, and non-citrus juices like apple juice or pear juice.
- Benefit: Decreases stomach acidity and minimizes reflux.

Caffeinated Drinks

- Swap: Coffee, black tea, and energy drinks.
- For: Herbal teas, decaffeinated coffee, and caffeine-free beverages.
- Benefit: Lowers stomach acid production.

Fried and Greasy Foods

- Swap: Fried chicken, french fries, and greasy fast food.
- For: Baked, grilled, or steamed options like baked chicken, roasted potatoes, and steamed vegetables.
- Benefit: Lowers fat intake and reduces reflux.

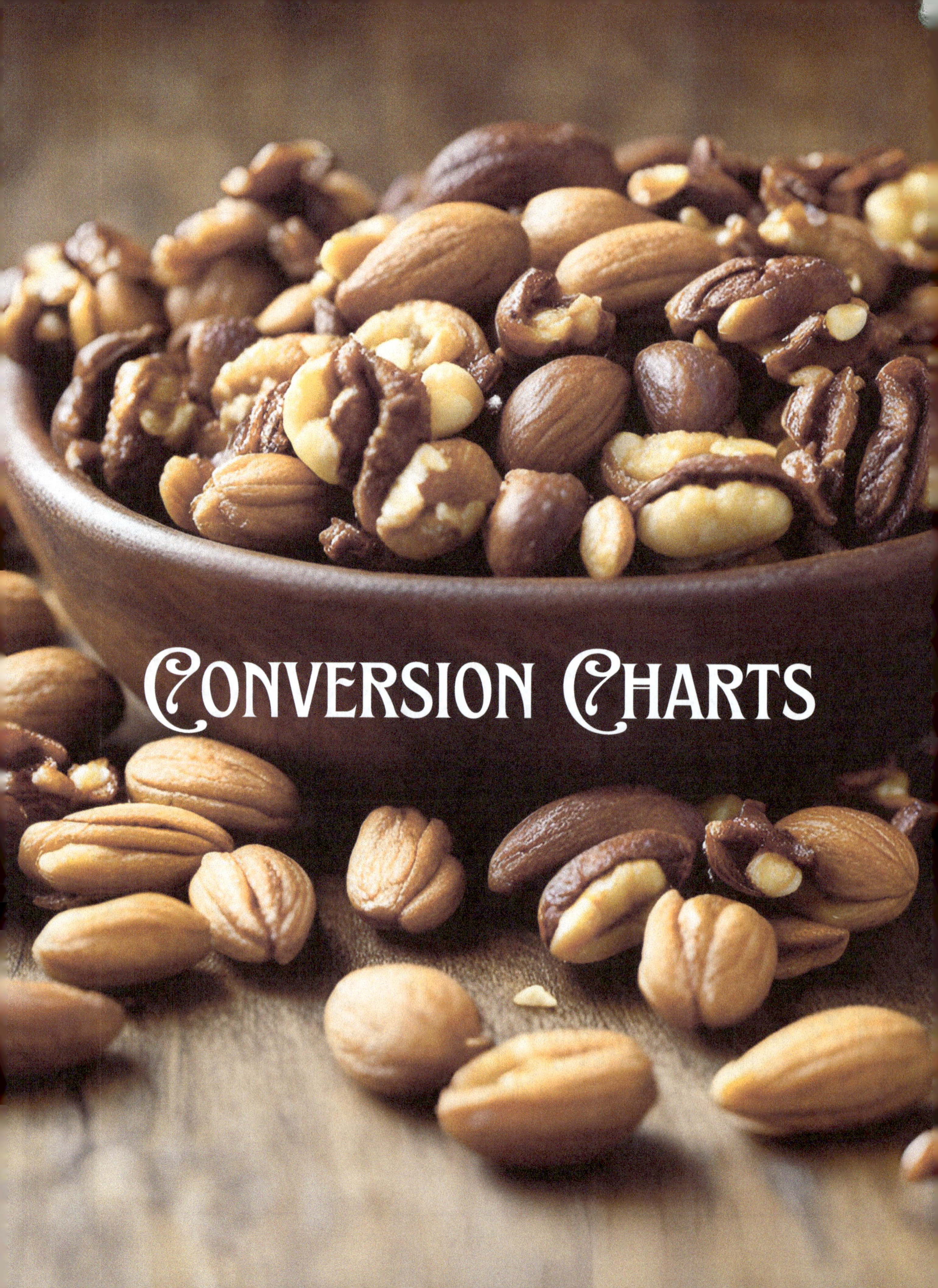

CONVERSION CHARTS

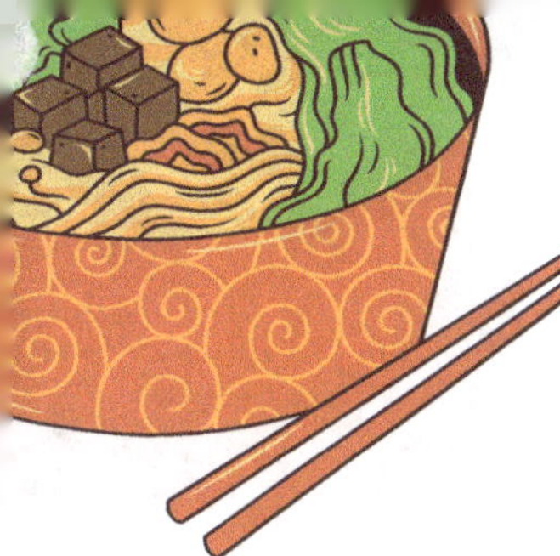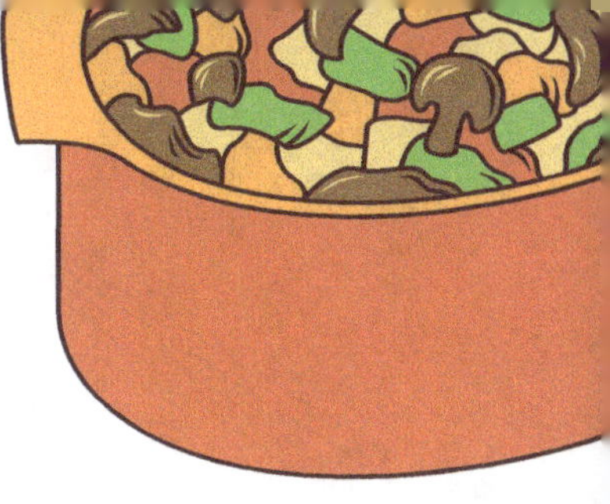

COMMON COOKING MEASUREMENTS

Volume Measurements

MEASUREMENT	EQUIVALENT
1 teaspoon (tsp)	1/3 tablespoon (tbsp)
1 teaspoon (tsp)	3 teaspoons (tsp)
1/8 cup	2 tablespoons (tbsp)
1/4 cup	4 tablespoons (tbsp)
1/3 cup	5 tablespoons + 1 teaspoon
1/2 cup	8 tablespoons (tbsp)
3/4 cup	12 tablespoons (tbsp)
1 cup	16 tablespoons (tbsp)
1 pint (pt)	2 cups
1 quart (qt)	4 cups
1 gallon (gal)	16 cups

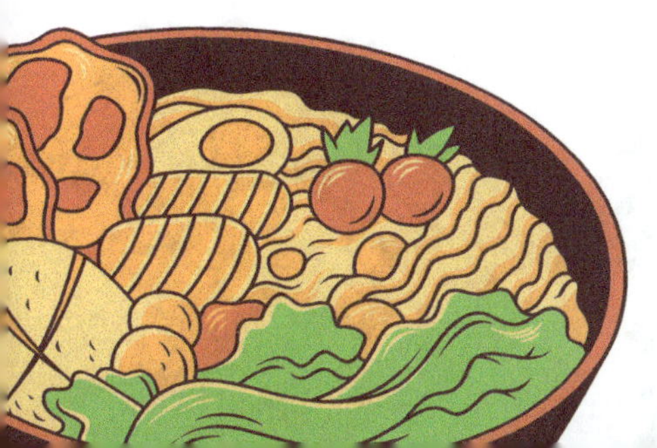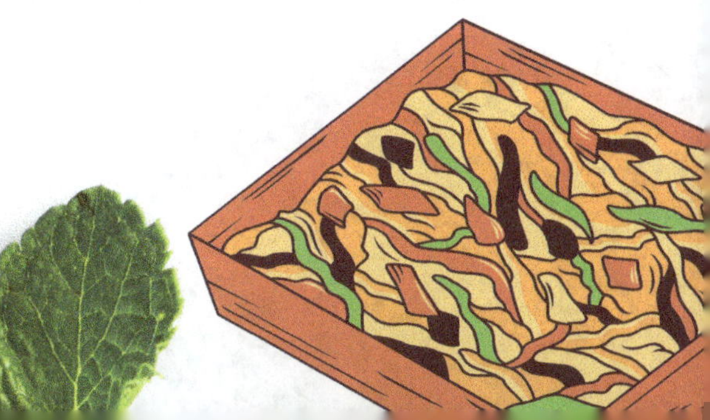

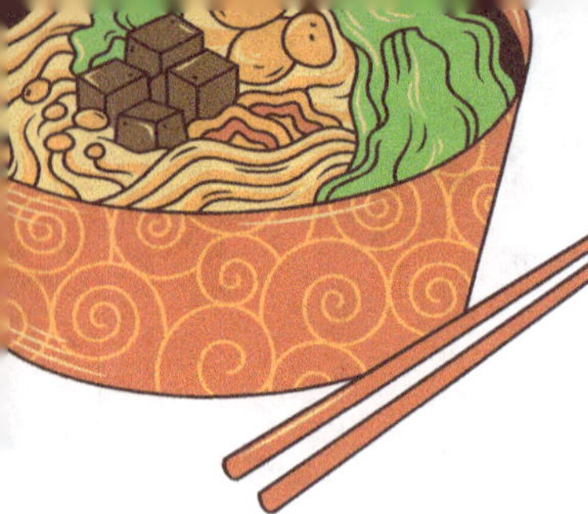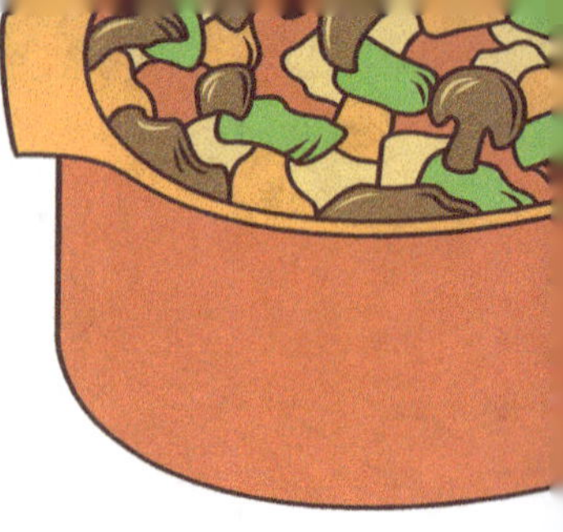

COMMON COOKING MEASUREMENTS

Weight Measurements

MEASUREMENT	EQUIVALENT
1 ounce (oz)	28.35 grams (g)
1 pound (lb)	16 ounces (oz)
1 kilogram (kg)	2.2 pounds (lbs)

Liquid Measurements

MEASUREMENT	EQUIVALENT
1 fluid ounce (fl oz)	2 tablespoons (tbsp)
1 cup	8 fluid ounces (fl oz)
1 pint (pt)	16 fluid ounces (fl oz)
1 quart (qt)	32 fluid ounces (fl oz)
1 gallon (gal)	128 fluid ounces (fl oz)

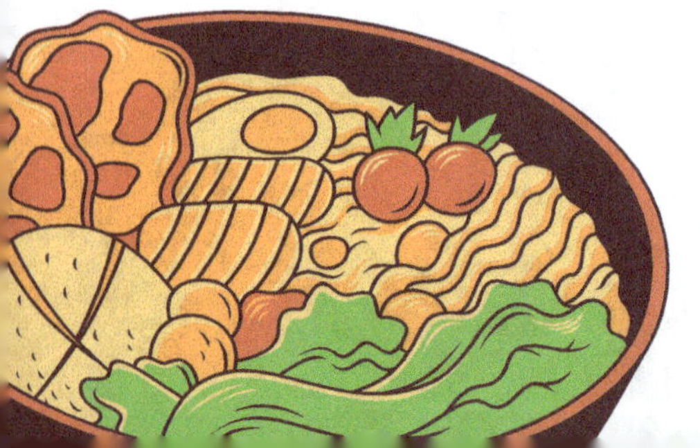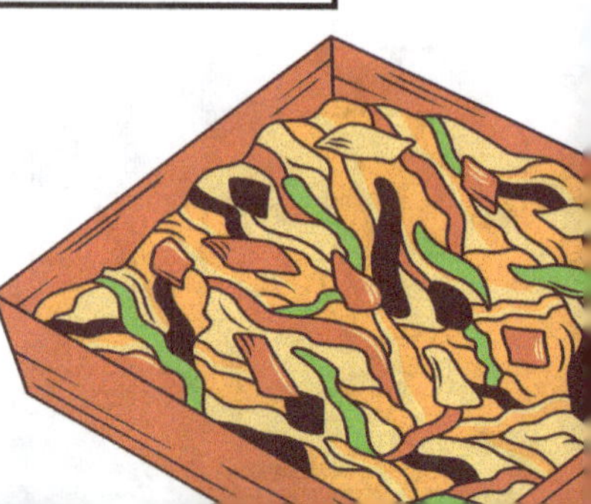

OVEN TEMPERATURES

Temperature Conversions

FAHRENHEIT (°F)	CELSIUS (°C)	GAS MARK
250°F	120°C	1/2
275°F	135°C	1
300°F	150°C	2
325°F	165°C	3
350°F	175°C	4
375°F	190°C	5
400°F	200°C	6
425°F	220°C	7
450°F	230°C	8
475°F	245°C	9
500°F	260°C	10

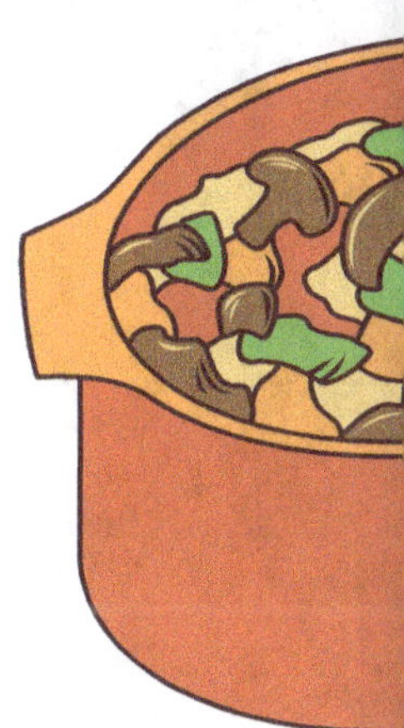

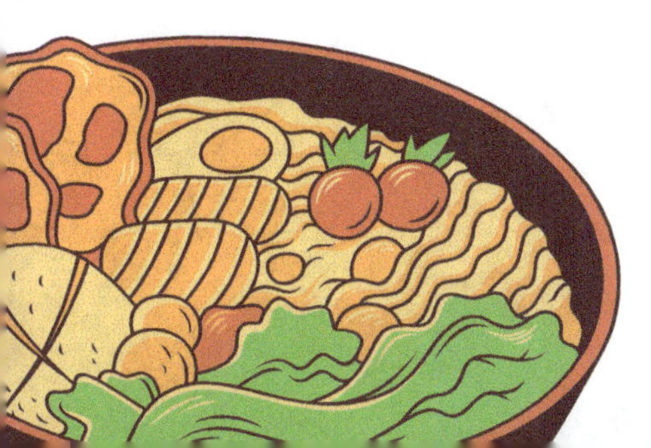

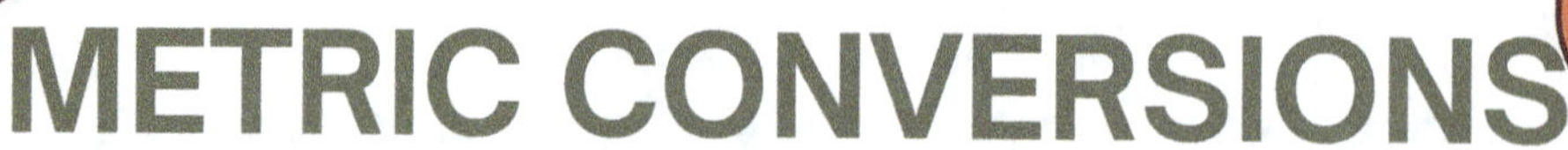

METRIC CONVERSIONS

Volume

METRIC	U.S. EQUIVALENT
1 milliliter (ml)	0.034 fluid ounces (fl oz)
100 milliliters	3.4 fluid ounces (fl oz)
1 liter (l)	34 fluid ounces (fl oz)
1 liter (l)	4.2 cups
1 liter (l)	2.1 pints

Weight

METRIC	U.S. EQUIVALENT
1 gram (g)	0.035 ounces (oz)
100 grams (g)	3.5 ounces (oz)
500 grams (g)	17.6 ounces (oz)
1 kilogram (kg)	2.2 pounds (lbs)

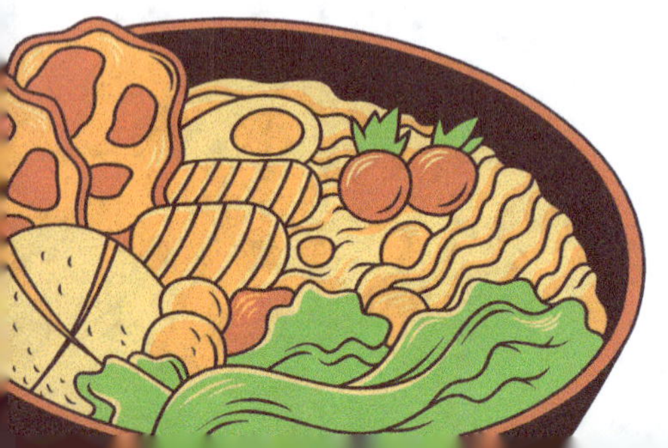
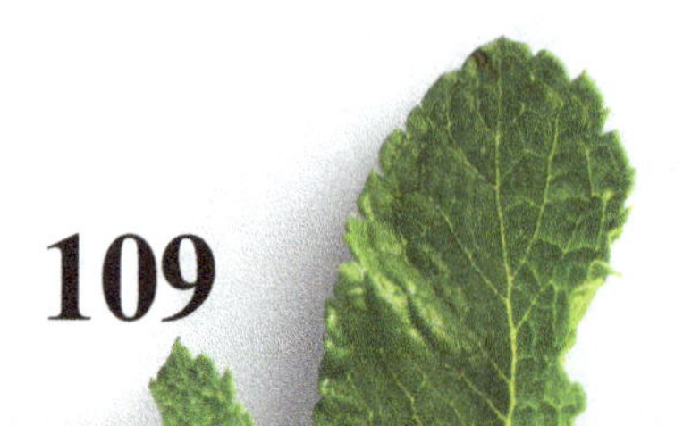
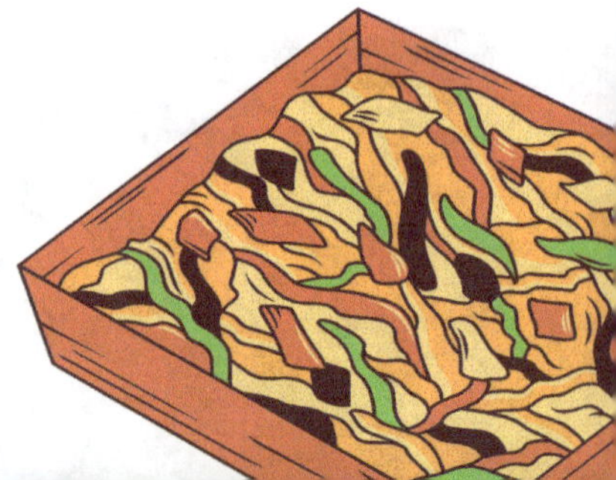

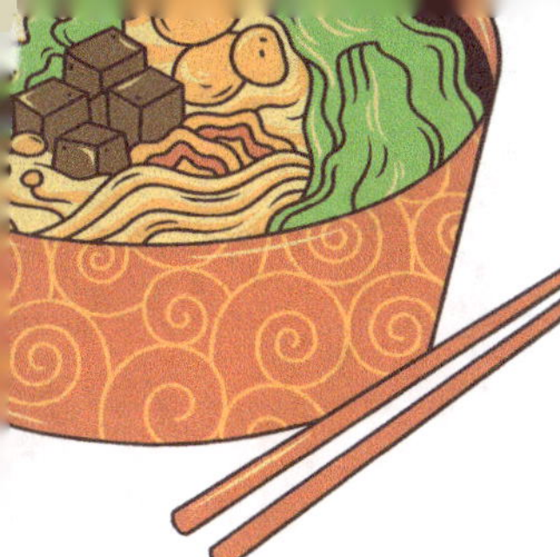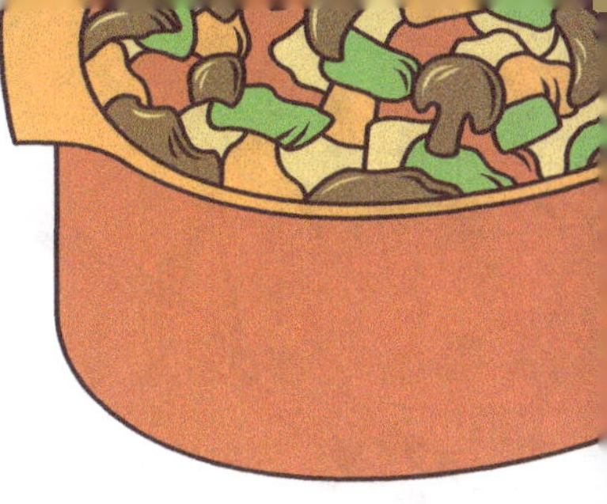

COMMON COOKING MEASUREMENTS

Volume Measurements

MEASUREMENT	EQUIVALENT
tsp	teaspoon
tbsp	tablespoon
Cup	Cup
oz	ounce
lb	pound
ml	milliliter
l	liter
g	gram
Kg	Kilogram
fl oz	fluid ounce

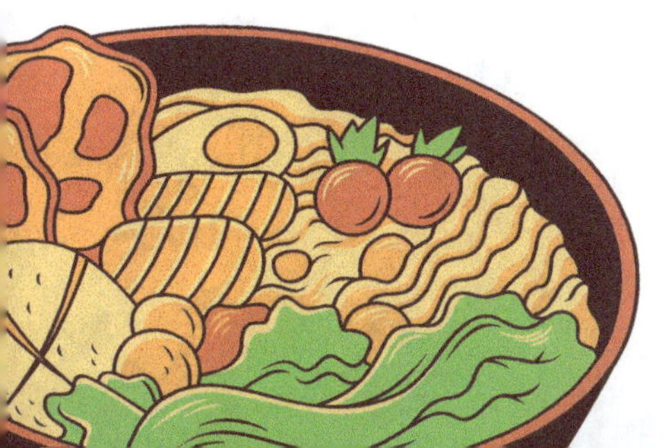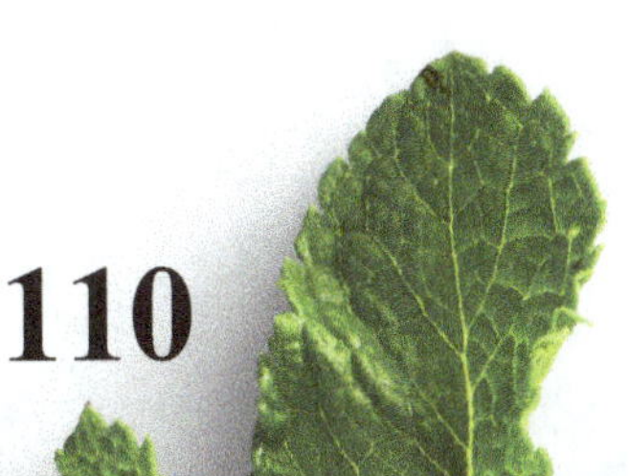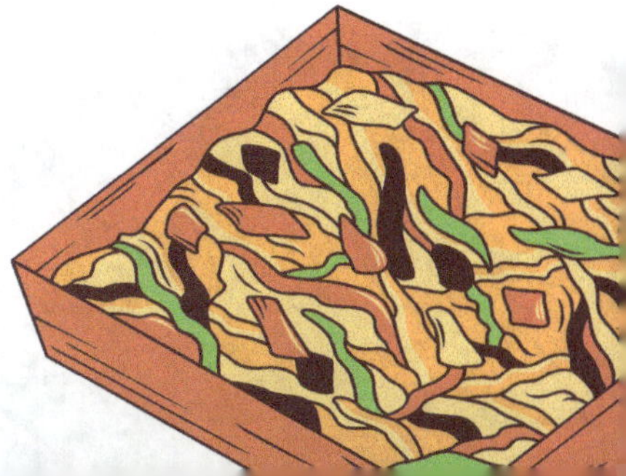

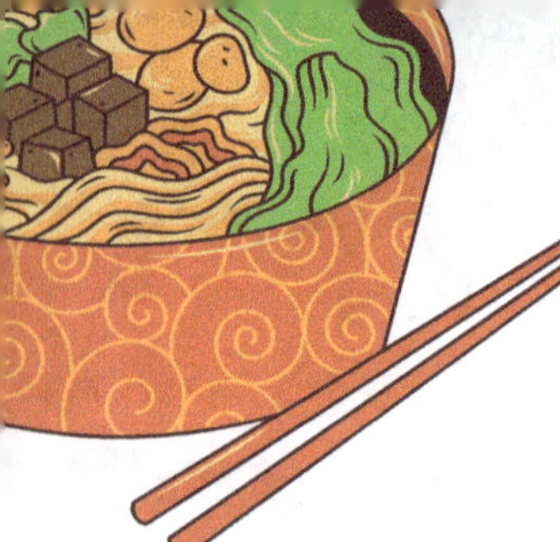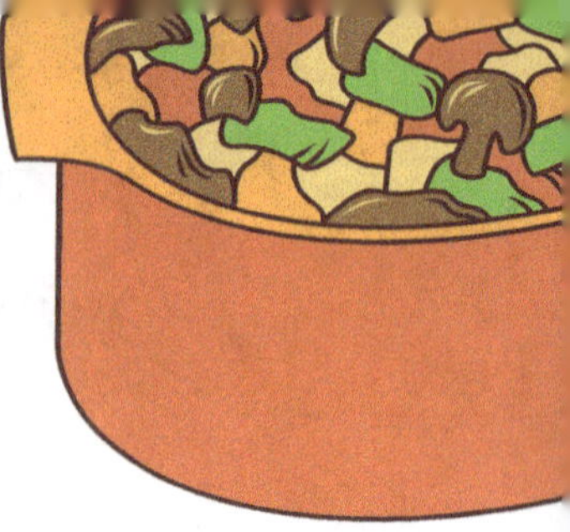

COMMON COOKING MEASUREMENTS

Volume Measurements

1 cup all-purpose flour = 120 grams
1 cup granulated sugar = 200 grams
1 cup brown sugar = 220 grams
1 cup butter = 227 grams (or 2 sticks)
1 large egg = 50 grams

Note:

- When measuring dry ingredients, use a spoon to fill the measuring cup or spoon, and level off with a flat edge for accuracy.
- For liquid ingredients, use a clear measuring cup and check at eye level.
- When converting recipes, be mindful of the precision required for baking versus cooking.

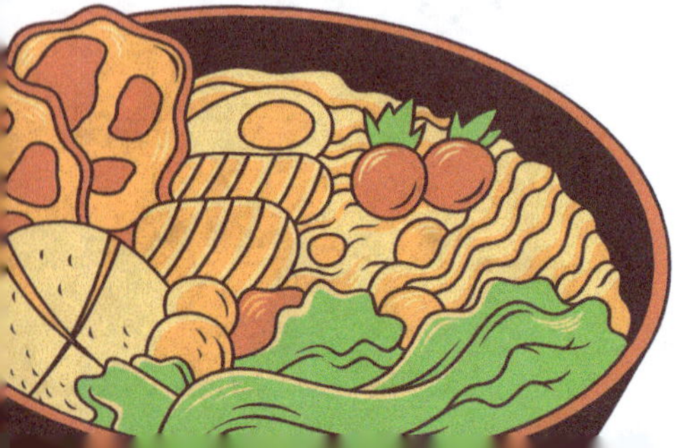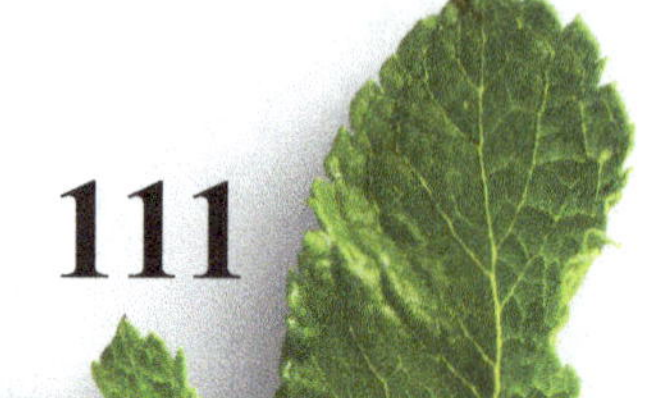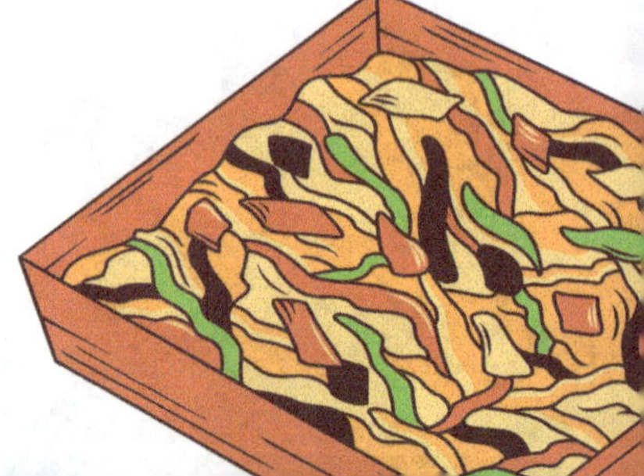

Conclusion

The journey to managing GERD through diet is one of patience, understanding, and making mindful choices. This cookbook, "GERD Diet Cookbook for Beginners," has provided a comprehensive guide to navigating this path with confidence and creativity. From understanding the fundamentals of GERD and its triggers to mastering the art of preparing delicious, GERD-friendly meals, you now have the tools to make dietary decisions that support your health and well-being.

Adopting a GERD-friendly diet involves more than just changing the foods you eat; it's about embracing a lifestyle that prioritizes your digestive health. The recipes and tips provided in this cookbook are designed to help you enjoy a variety of flavors and cuisines while minimizing discomfort. By making smart food swaps, planning meals ahead, and using batch cooking techniques, you can create a sustainable eating pattern that supports your digestive system.

Managing GERD is a continuous journey that requires awareness and adaptability. By keeping a food diary, you can track your triggers and make informed decisions about what to eat. Remember, it's not about deprivation but about finding and enjoying the foods that make you feel your best.

As you move forward, continue to experiment with new recipes and ingredients, always paying attention to how your body responds. Share your successes and challenges with your healthcare provider to fine-tune your diet and ensure it meets your nutritional needs.

Thank you for choosing the "GERD Diet Cookbook for Beginners" as your guide. We hope it serves as a valuable resource in your journey to better health. Remember, with the right knowledge and tools, you can manage GERD effectively and enjoy a fulfilling, delicious, and symptom-free life.

Living with GERD doesn't mean you have to sacrifice flavor or enjoyment in your meals. With the recipes and strategies provided in this cookbook, you are well-equipped to make dietary choices that support your digestive health. Here's to a healthier, happier you—one meal at a time. Bon appétit!

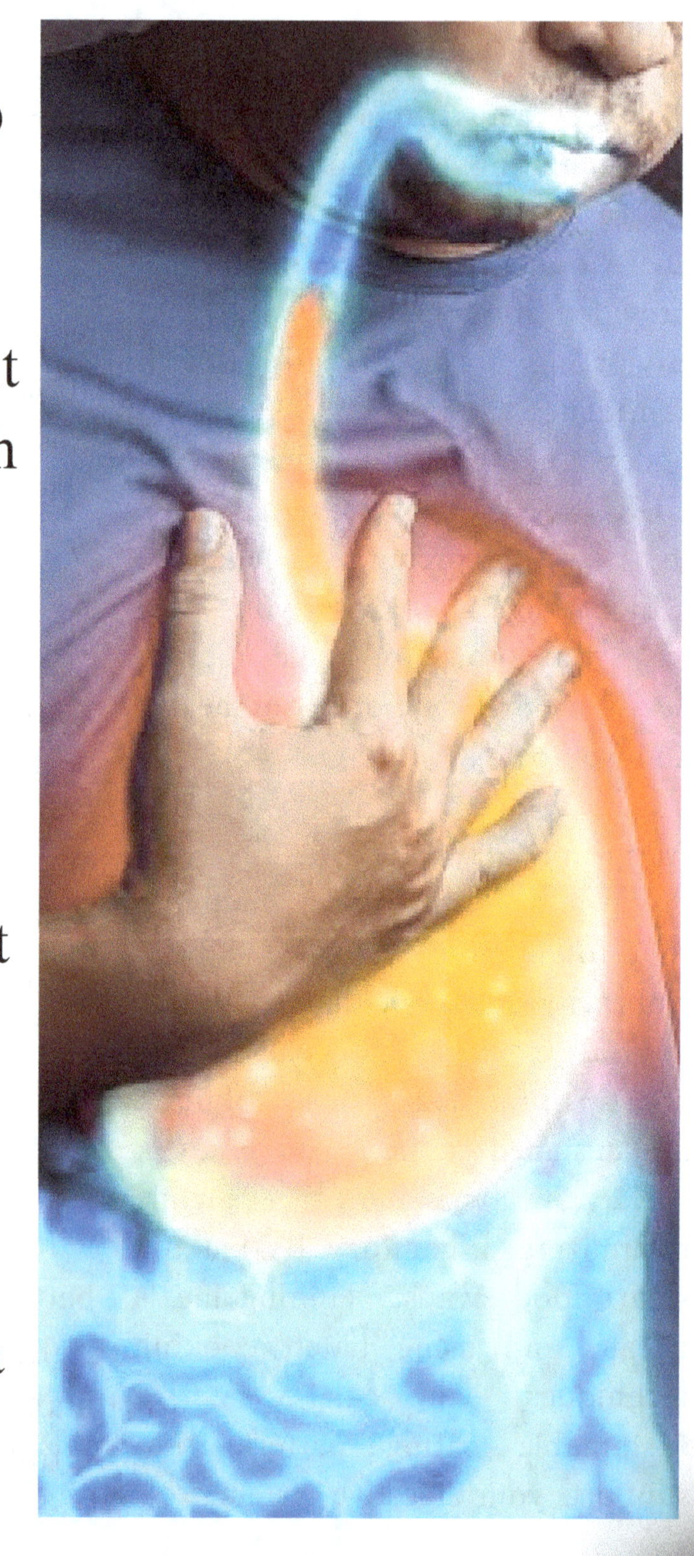

DISCOVER MORE ABOUT MY CULINARY ADVENTURES AND UPCOMING PROJECTS.

THE AUTHOR

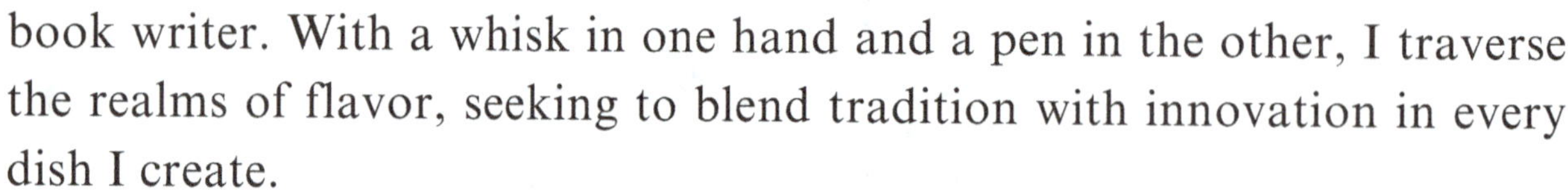

Hello, culinary adventurers!
I'm Vakare Rimkute, a passionate explorer of the culinary world and a devoted recipe book writer. With a whisk in one hand and a pen in the other, I traverse the realms of flavor, seeking to blend tradition with innovation in every dish I create.

Growing up in the bustling kitchens of my Lithuanian grandmother, I developed an insatiable curiosity for the alchemy of ingredients and the magic they could weave on the palate. From the rustic charm of hearty stews to the delicate intricacies of pastries, my journey through food has been nothing short of a delightful adventure.

After years of experimenting and honing my craft, I found my true calling as a recipe book writer. With each recipe I pen, I aim to capture the essence of culinary culture while infusing it with a touch of modern flair. From comforting classics to bold culinary experiments, my recipes are a reflection of my belief that food should not only nourish the body but also nourish the soul.

So join me on this gastronomic journey, where every page is filled with tantalizing flavors, heartwarming stories, and a dash of humor. Together, let's embark on a culinary adventure that will tickle your taste buds and leave you craving for more. Happy cooking!